SECRETS
of
GORGEOUS

Hundreds of Ways to Live Well
While Living It Up

Esther Blum, M.S., R.D., C.D.N., C.N.S.

CHRONICLE BOOKS
SAN FRANCISCO

Library of Congress Cataloging-in-Publication
Data:

Blum, Esther.
 Secrets of gorgeous : hundreds of ways to live
well while living it up / by Esther Blum.
  p. cm.
 Includes index.
 ISBN: 978-0-8118-6581-4
 1. Nutrition. 2. Beauty, Personal. I. Title.

 RA784.B5582 2008
 612.3--dc22

                          2008010491
Printed in China

Design by Jay Peter Salvas

10 9 8 7 6 5 4 3

Chronicle Books LLC
680 Second Street
San Francisco, California 94107

www.chroniclebooks.com

For BENJAMIN, my son-shine.

CONTENTS

INTRODUCTION

Remember, Ginger Rogers did everything Fred Astaire did, but backwards and in high heels. — Faith Whittlesey

The best gifts come in small packages. My last book, *Eat, Drink, and Be Gorgeous,* was about living well while living it up. The book you now hold in your hands is a continuation on that theme—the must-have little Pink Bible of lifestyle to open up and flip through when you need some divine inspiration. Think of it as a clutch-sized accessory for the gorgeous lady on the go. It's chock-full of my best secrets and tips on being gorgeous inside and out.

Before we get to the tips, I'd like to say a few words about being gorgeous. The very essence of being gorgeous isn't about being perfect: It's about being and feeling our most fabulous. And the secret of doing that is accepting your imperfections; I prefer to think of these as attributes. As a nutritionist, I love to make my clients laugh about their perceived imperfections and inspire them to take responsibility for themselves. Rather than fight against the machine that rages inside of us, why not shift gears and go with the flow? A little self-acceptance goes a long way in softening our own critical voice, which can serve as a barrier to helping us reach our goals.

People often assume that because I am a nutritionist, I am somehow exempt from ever wanting or craving any kind of junk food. If I am out on the town and indulging in a martini or two, or my fave chocolate dessert, I have to be prepared for the reaction that inevitably comes my way, should I run into a patient. Some Gorgeous Girls are psyched that a nutritionist is validating their food choices in a very real way. Others may be appalled: *"Who is this woman who has the balls to tell me what to do and then goes and eats a jumbo M&M-studded cookie?!"* This makes my message to you all the more heartfelt. Eating cookies is a very real part of who I am and who I will always be. I'd love to think I could be a yogi eating air all day, gaining strength from all my willpower and inner peace. But my relationship with chocolate goes *deep,* and I have to accept that this is me. By accepting this truth, I set myself free from the pressures of the world to do yet one more thing perfectly, and then I can move on with my life. . . . Until the next time I bake cookies, that is.

The tips in this little gem of a book will help you to become your own detective and find what works for *you.* You'll learn how food affects your body's digestive system, weight, energy levels, and gorgeous glow.

You'll also learn that the tips in this book are not one-size-fits-all. For more than fifteen years I have been going to nutrition and medical conferences. I've attended countless roundtable discussions on epidemiological studies, and guess what? The only thing experts ever seem to agree upon is that there is no one diet for everyone. Every gal's DNA is unique, like snowflakes, so how can we expect that diets are a one-size-fits-all remedy? When I work with patients it never ceases to amaze me how different people respond to the same foods. Some vegetarians, for example, gain weight when they increase protein intake and decrease carbohydrates, while more carnivorous types pack on the pounds when they even so much as glance at a grain of rice! So keep an open mind as you try the tips in this book. Some may work like a charm, others may be better for your sister or best girlfriend.

You'll find chapters here on everything from eating gorgeous to drinking gorgeous to, my favorite, being gorgeous in bed. These days, it seems like wooing a man with our God-given womanly charm just isn't good enough. Advertisers do all they can to convince us that we've got to get waxed, shaved, and plucked beforehand; we need to look, taste, and smell great; and to top it all, we have to perform well. In other words, the pressure is on. It's enough to give a girl a complex. So when pesky problems like vaginal dryness or a bum libido make an uninvited appearance, they can really cramp your style. The good news is that nutrition once again comes to the rescue. No, it can't give you Pamela Anderson breasts or a J. Lo booty. But nutrition can get your motor running and help you take entertaining at home to a whole new level.

The chapter on being gorgeously fit will give you loads of tips on how to challenge yourself. I've made a point to offer lots of great exercise ideas so you can incorporate new types of fitness into your regime. The Gorgeous in Green chapter proves that being eco-conscious has never been sexier or more important. Companies are finally jumping on the bandwagon, and a slow but sure paradigm shift is taking place.

Call me ever optimistic, but I feel that increasing folks' green awareness alters the way we think about Mama Earth and our relationship with her. Green products not only preserve the environment, but using them also gives our bodies a break from the hard work of first metabolizing, then detoxifying from, the harsh chemicals present in the majority of non-green products. I don't know about you, but the only time I want to spend laid up in bed is when I'm getting laid!

The thing to remember about being gorgeous is this: We are responsible for change on both a personal and a global level. The voice of one is mighty; factor in the voice of each and every one of us, and you will see that we *can* move mountains together. Want to reduce dependence on foreign oil, and oil in general, while getting healthy? Switch to glass bottles. Want to go natural even when you're naked? Try some organic lube. Positive energy and action in the name of green is all good.

We all have unlimited strength and beauty within ourselves. I hope that in reading this book, you feel inspired to make a few small changes here and there that can make huge differences in how you feel and how you glow. I also hope *Secrets of Gorgeous* serves as a reminder that being healthy can be loads of fun and should be a huge part of your life.

STAY GORGEOUS,
Esther

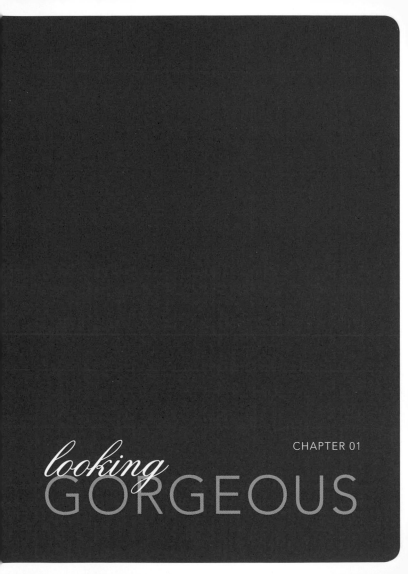

CHAPTER 01

looking
GORGEOUS

skin deep: NATURAL FACE-LIFT

Our skin is our greatest accessory; a glowing complexion is worth far more than any item of clothing and/or any compact of makeup you will ever buy. Always nourish your skin with nutritious, whole foods, and keep sugar use on the low end. Sugar causes all sorts of inflammation, including acne, and can leave you looking far older than your years if you eat too much of it; so indulge in high-quality treats on occasion but leave it at that. Here are my top tips for foods to firm the face:

- Eat wild Alaskan salmon at least three times per week; it's a face-lift in your fridge.
- Eat avocado and raw nuts and seeds to moisturize your skin from within.
- Eat blueberries and cantaloupe to plump up and protect the delicate cells of your skin that help you look beautiful.
- Drink green tea and lots of water each day.
- Most importantly, love the skin you're in and take good care of it—it's the only skin you've got!

skin deep: FISH FACE

Eating plenty of wild Alaskan salmon will help keep you gorgeous, since it contains astaxanthin and DMAE. Astaxanthin is the red algae that salmon eat, which gives them their pink color; it acts as both a natural sunscreen and a wrinkle-fighter. DMAE, a derivative of choline called dimethylaminoethanol, gives contours to your face and body by stimulating your muscles to contract under your skin. Think of it as your internal plastic surgeon. Plus, DMAE is great for the brain and helps improve cognitive function.

skin deep: TOPICAL TOXINS

To treat your skin and body kindly, use only the most natural products available. Steer clear of the following substances and read labels closely:

1. Synthetic colors like FD&C or D&C—all are potential carcinogens

2. Talc—a mineral that has been linked to respiratory damage

3. Dibutyl phthalate—a hormone-disrupting chemical

4. DMDM hydantoin quaternium-15 and diazonlidnyl urea—formaldehyde-releasing preservatives

5. Parabens—butyl-, ethyl-, methyl-, and propyl-parabens mimic estrogen and may result in reproductive damage

skin deep: POLISHED TO PERFECTION

To exfoliate your face: Apply a dime-sized amount of plain sugar to your wet face (steer clear of the eye area) in tiny circular motions until the sugar turns into a sticky serum (up to three minutes) and watch it work wonders! Rinse off with warm water and apply the healing moisturizer of your choice. Look at that lovely glow!

skin deep: GOODBYE, CELLULITE!

Trying to eliminate cellulite isn't just about vanity, it's also about health. Cellulite is a sign that your inner detoxification pathways have a wrench in the works. It may be a metabolic issue, it may be a dietary issue. Either way, it's possible to get to the root of the problem and smooth out its appearance.

First and foremost, stop smoking. Cigarettes damage vein and capillary walls, making them inflamed and leaky. Nicotine constricts blood vessels, which narrows our delicate internal pipes, meaning less nutrients go in, less toxins get out, then boom—a cesspool of stagnant yuck on your innards and thighs.

Lymphatic drainage, the equivalent of putting Drano in a clogged pipe, is a powerful tool in the war against cellulite. It gets your circulation going and facilitates the removal of waste products and toxins. It's easy, too. Deep breathing (think yoga) increases blood and lymph flow and will drench your skin cells with nutrients and oxygen. Massage also stimulates the cleansing flow of the lymphatic vessels.

Jumping rope or rebounding on a trampoline are great fat-busters that are effective in as little as five minutes per day. Regular exercise, especially interval training, is another great route to take. Not only will it increase circulation, it will also bust up fat in the deeper layers of the skin and build muscle to decrease the jiggles.

skin deep: FEEL THE RUSH WITH A SKIN BRUSH

For those Gorgeous Gals who'd love a daily detox, here's a non-invasive, calorie-burning, cheap way to get it: daily skin brushing. Skin brushing removes dead skin cells and clears space for your pores to get rid of your internal junk. Brushing removes impurities from the body and promotes lymphatic drainage, which helps reduce the appearance of cellulite—yippee!

Here's the best way to dry brush: Purchase a long-handled soft-bristled brush or loofah. Before you shower or take a bath, start by brushing your feet, then work up to the legs, your booty, your abdomen, and chest (go easy on the breasts!). Always brush from the back towards the heart. Brush every morning to get your lymphatic system stimulated and your skin glowing. This is one of the simplest and effective ways to change the appearance of your dimpled areas. Buh-bye lumpy and dumpy. Hello smooth and sexy.

skin deep: YOU'RE SO VEIN

Spider or varicose veins are pesky problems caused by many factors, like standing all day, always sitting cross-legged, a pregnancy, or plain old genetic predisposition. They result from vascular integrity loss and are almost always associated with liver congestion. Although standing on your feet all day won't cause liver congestion, it can exacerbate an underlying problem that already exists. The good news is that cleaning up your liver (also see Liver Detox, page 179) to increase circulation also helps your body detox on a daily basis. Liver detox also improves your digestion and energy levels, and even potentially prevents hangovers.

Vein Therapy

- **Collinsonia root (stone root):** Collinsonia has been proven to help clear out stubborn varicose veins (and hemorrhoids, too!). Give yourself 6 to 12 weeks to see results. Take 4 to 6 capsules per day with a full glass of water.
- **A-F betafood:** A whole-food supplement derived from beetroot and carrots, A-F betafood helps support liver function and fats' breakdown. Take 6 tablets per day.
- **Milk thistle:** Take 300 mg per day.

If you love to show off your gams but the roadmap on the backs of your legs is off-putting, you can always cover up your veins with makeup or self-tanner.

skin deep: WART THWART

Warts are stubborn little guys that dig in deep and just don't quit. To get rid of them, you've got to work aggressively and fast. If you've tried unsuccessfully to give them the old heave-ho using traditional methods (freezing, topical treatments), give this natural remedy a whirl. It will cost you pennies at most, and your wart should be gone in four to eight weeks, depending on its size.

Pick up a bottle of unpasteurized organic apple cider vinegar. Each night before bed, soak the infected area in warm water for about 15 minutes. Remove the cotton from the end of a Q-tip and dip it into the raw organic apple cider vinegar. Secure the saturated cotton to the wart with a bandage, and leave it on overnight. Repeat every night until the wart turns dark brown and peels off.

nails: CUTE-ICLES

If your cuticles resemble crusty little craters crying out for hydration, look no further than the aisles of your local drugstore. Aquaphor is an easy, at-home remedy that will not only heal your hands but will save you tons of money at the manicurists.

Every morning and evening, grab some Aquaphor and massage a dab into your cuticles. Aquaphor is also great for chapped lips; dry, cracked heels; and preventing chafing during all sorts of athletic endurance events (think butt cheeks rubbing together during a long run).

Gorgeous Girl beware! One endurance activity for which Aquaphor should NOT be used is sex. It's way too thick to be a lubricant, and even worse, it decreases the efficacy of latex. No Gorgeous Girl wants that!

nails: NAIL DOWN THE ISSUE

Whether you love yourself some long, colorful talons or prefer short and sassy nippers, every gal wants lovely, healthy nails. Not only do nails tell a story about how a gal cares for her outsides, they also reveal a lot about how she cares for her insides. Nails are often the first thing I, as a nutritionist, examine on a person. So let's size you up first, and then I'll tell you what nutrients will help correct any issues:

PROBLEM	SOLUTION
Soft nails that tear or peel easily	Pump more protein into your diet
Dry, brittle nails that break easily	Add calcium-rich foods and supplements
Horizontal or vertical ridges	Get your thyroid checked
Thin, flat, spoon-shaped nail beds	Check your iron levels and grab a steak plus supplemental iron if necessary
White spots on nails or nail bed	Think zinc
Darkened nail beds	Add B_{12} supplements

nails: GIVE THEM A BREATHER

I love it when clients moon me—not *that* kind of mooning. White moons at the cuticle reveal the levels of antioxidants in the body. So if you can't spy any white at the cuticle, start taking supplements rich in antioxidants (especially vitamin E). If you have poor circulation, you'll exhibit any of the symptoms on page 21. And don't be afraid to go naked and bare for a sexy change of pace. Excessive exposure to nail polish, nail polish remover, plus any type of chemical solvent also causes dry, brittle nails.

hair: TO DYE FOR

Although I currently don't color my curls, I know I'll run to my hairy godmother the minute I spy a lick of gray. So, to be prepared when that time comes, I wanted to figure out my options now. Loving the concept of going au naturel, I was curious to see if natural hair dye wasn't just an oxymoron.

Here's what I learned: It's tough to know how much of the harmful chemicals in hair dyes gets absorbed into our bodies. Peroxide and ammonia may not be carcinogenic, but they can be very dangerous to those with chemical sensitivities. And permanent hair dyes contain petrochemicals, which are derived from petroleum and are used to manufacture plastics. On the flip side, there are natural colors out there that are less damaging to hair and less toxic to the body, but with fewer chemicals comes less coverage.

What's the happy medium? Look for dyes free of PPD (para-phenylenediamine), which is a known carcinogen. And look into semipermanent color, which is ammonia-free. For all you real blondies out there, henna takes out the gray but won't lighten your hair. For lighter locks grab some lemons, spritz the juice on your hair, and go soak up some sunshine!

hair removal:

PERFECTION FROM A CONFECTION

If your skin is sensitive or you are prone to breakouts or allergic reactions, all-natural wax can help reduce skin irritation and unsightly red bumps and itching. Wax containing aloe (usually tinted blue) also helps ease discomfort. If you'd like to go completely natural and chemical-free when it comes to hair removal, consider sugaring. Sugaring is the exact same concept as waxing, but instead of removing hair with wax, the hair is removed with a sugaring paste. Sugaring paste is made primarily of sugar. It is completely natural and gentle on the skin and is easily cleaned up with water. The results can be as effective as waxing, too. Sugaring paste can be used anywhere you'd normally use wax for a silky smooth you that's even sweeter than before! For you adventuresome types, try this with an at-home kit, but for the rest of you less-nimble creatures, let someone else do the dirty work.

eyes: DECODING DARK CIRCLES

So you went on a bit of a bender last night, bar-hopping until the wee hours of the morning. Or even worse, you put in long hours at the office in front of the computer screen and your eyes are bleary and weary. Obviously, getting good-quality restful sleep is the number one antidote to unsightly under-eye circles. But if you're getting good sleep and haven't been overdoing it, your under-eye circles may indicate allergies. Blue under-eye circles are related to food allergies, especially dairy products. Try eliminating dairy for four months to give your immune and digestive systems a rest, and you should see a positive difference in your blue moons. If your under-eye circles are downtown brown, that is a sign of liver stress. This is a good time to reassess your coffee, cigarette, and booze intake. Incorporate shots of wheatgrass and dark green leafy vegetables into your diet, and take 300 mg of milk thistle per day.

feet: SEXY SHOES AND SEXY FEET

Every gorgeous gal knows that shoes are the most important wardrobe decision you make, so choose and invest wisely, because funky deformities like hammer toes, bunions, and calluses are a far cry from sexy. For Gorgeous Girls who are loathe to give up their towering heels for comfort, I'm here to tell you you can have your stilettos and wear them, too.

SHOE-DO'S

So what's a gal to do when she's rushing about town in pointy-toe stilettos with no time to rest her weary tootsies?

- Make sure your heel doesn't ride up and down when you walk. Save riding up and down for the bedroom. Stilettos optional.
- When shopping, try your shoes on at day's end, when your feet tend to be the most swollen.
- Natural materials like leather or canvas are much more forgiving than a man-made material.
- Size does matter! Fit your shoes to accommodate your largest foot, as your feet aren't equally matched in size. Make sure you have enough wiggle room in the toe area.
- My favorite stiletto secret? Dr. Scholl's insoles—slide them into your heels for extra comfort. Also give your dogs an occasional rest. Every day or two slip on some sassy flats and channel Audrey Hepburn.

feet: TREAT YOUR TOOTSIES

Are your tootsies feeling achy, tired, and crabby? Wash the day's fatigue off your feet with an aromatherapy foot soak:

½ cup **Epsom salts**
1 teaspoon **baking soda**
2 drops **essential oil of lemon**
2 drops **essential oil of sandalwood**
2 drops **essential oil of coriander**

Mix the ingredients well in warm water in a foot basin or bathtub with enough water to immerse your feet up to your ankles. (If you really need a body soak at day's end, feel free to immerse your whole self in the tub, but quadruple the recipe for best results.) Soak for 15 minutes. Ah, what bliss . . .

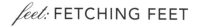 *feel:* FETCHING FEET

If the bottoms of your feet look like a cross between crusty molten lava and crusty old bread (you ladies know who you are!), get to work with this Sugar Scrub. It will gently and effectively erase telltale signs of wear and tear so you can go bare with confidence! The key to this scrub is to make it fresh. Don't let it sit longer than a week.

Sugar Scrub

¼–½ cup **sugar**
1–2 tablespoons **extra virgin olive oil**
    (more or less, as desired)
2 drops **essential oil of lavender**, or any other
    essential oil of your choice

Place the sugar in a Tupperware container, then pour in the extra virgin olive oil to moisturize the sugar. (You may need to add in a little extra oil, depending on desired consistency.) Add in two drops of the essential oil.

Next, bust out your pumice and scrub-a-dub-dub your problem spots until the sugar dissolves and the scrub turns into a serum—this is where glycolic acid comes from, which is actually a wonderful exfoliant for the skin. (Finally, sugar is good for something!) Rinse and dab dry. Voilà!

feet: ATHLETE'S FOOT

The greatest irony of athlete's foot is that it often has nothing to do with being an athlete. Wearing übersnug Chucks or walking barefoot in public locker rooms, gyms, or indoor pool areas can all contribute to the cause.

To treat athlete's foot, make sure you thoroughly dry your feet after showering—especially between the toes. Air out your feet in open shoes; moisture and heat combined are a foot's worst enemy. Shake a little powder between your toes, and don't go barefoot in public (except at the beach).

Topically, apply tea tree oil to the affected areas. Tea tree oil is an antiseptic and kills many bacteria and fungi. For best results, apply a 50 percent tea tree oil solution twice daily to the funky areas. After four weeks you should see a marked improvement. Toeriffic!

feel: FOOTLOOSE AND FUNGUS-FREE

Is there anything worse in life than nail fungus? Not in sandal season! If you find yourself on the receiving end of the gift that keeps on giving, then you know what a drag it can be. Nail fungus is like that annoying guy who keeps hitting on you—very stubborn and very hard to get rid of. But I've learned that if you treat them both aggressively, they'll eventually get the message and disappear for good.

Best of all, there's no need for those costly, liver-damaging drugs. These home remedies are safe and cost-effective. Just be consistent, and apply twice a day, every day—no excuses.

- Mix a solution of one part tea tree oil and one part lavender oil. Take a Q-tip or brush and apply the oil to the entire infected nail and the area around it. Tea tree oil is a natural antibiotic and antiseptic, and lavender oil will fight the infection and prevent skin irritation, plus, it smells pretty.
- If you don't mind the smell of vinegar, use a medicine dropper and apply apple cider vinegar directly to the nail. Fungus cannot thrive in such an acidic environment, so the infection will soon die.
- No matter which solution you choose, apply religiously until the nail grows out completely; this could mean up to six months for fingernails, and up to twelve months for toenails. Stick with it!

teeth: HIGH GLOSS WITH FLOSS

This may sound crazy, but flossing daily can significantly strengthen your primary immune system. It's true. Regular flossing decreases your risk for heart disease, diabetes, osteoporosis, and respiratory infections all while freshening up your kisser. Consider it your dental fitness program. Flossing once per day, brushing twice per day, and visiting your dentist regularly are requisite steps in staying gorgeous from the inside out. How? Flossing and brushing get rid of the bad bacteria—the same bacteria that can lead to cardiovascular disease—that's hanging out in your mouth.

It's also best to use natural products for your oral hygiene. Look for toothpastes containing baking soda, sea salt, or calcium carbonate to remove plaque and polish teeth to perfection. Essential oils such as peppermint, cinnamon, and wintergreen stimulate gums and freshen your breath. Other ingredients such as propolis, myrrh, tea tree, and echinacea can help slow bacterial growth, strengthen gum tissue, and prevent inflammation. And if you are prone to periodontal diseases (such as gingivitis or receding gums) make sure you pop 200 mg of coenzyme Q10 (CoQ10) per day to heal up those gums straightaway.

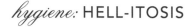

hygiene: HELL-ITOSIS

Halitosis is often caused by a buildup of bacteria in the mouth from food debris, plaque, gum disease, or a coating on the back of the tongue. Good oral hygiene will usually solve the problem. Keep up with regular brushing of your teeth and tongue, flossing, and using antiseptic mouthwash. And watch out for odiferous foods—if they smell to you, then they will smell to others! Garlic, onions, and sardines are just a few likely offenders.

Eating clean, fresh foods and cutting back on dairy will also fight bad breath, since dairy often produces extra mucus in the intestinal tract. If you notice your breath's not so fresh, then try cutting dairy out altogether for a month, and see if that works for you.

Be wary of junk foods in general—nobody ever improved their breath eating Doritos and Milk Duds! Your breath is a great barometer of your internal health, so if you're filling up your insides with junk, what you expel out to the world surely won't be any better. Turn yourself into a clean, green eating machine and say tootles to all things rank.

hygiene: SOMETHING WICKED THIS WAY COMES

Have you ever discreetly lifted up your arm to sniff your pits, only to discover that your natural scent has been edged out by Eau de Roadkill? If you suffer from stinky underarms, try a natural deodorant containing tea tree oil or baking soda. Tea tree oil has antibacterial properties, and baking soda also mops up bad odors.

To be stench-free from within, think about supporting your liver. Before you give me the stink-eye, keep in mind that most body odor emanates from a congested liver or one that detoxifies poorly. So be sure to eat enough protein (supports liver function and metabolizes hormones) and dark green leafy vegetables, and pop 300 mg of milk thistle per day.

travel: WANDERLUST MUSTS

Traveling today sure isn't as glamorous as it used to be. But there are several ways to stay gorgeous in the air or on the road:

- Bring a small carry-on with these essential picks: a sleep mask to help melatonin production and encourage peaceful slumber; moisturizer for the face and hands to combat the dry, recycled air; as much water as possible; sumptuous snacks like raw nuts and seeds, goji berries, crackers and cheese, and fresh fruit; a cashmere scarf (this also doubles as a blanket); relaxing reading materials; and earplugs or an MP3 player.
- To protect your skin and body from the dry, recycled air, be sure to take antioxidants both before and during the flight. This will also help you fight airborne bugs from other passengers and recover more quickly from jet lag.
- Lastly, don't forget to get up and stretch at least once an hour to promote circulation and prevent swollen, puffy feet.

SUPPLEMENTS TO RULE THE SKIES

Vitamin C	500 mg before the flight and 500 mg midflight
Wheatgrass powder	Reconstitute with water for a refreshingly delish mocktail
Green tea	Also a great in-flight beverage that is saturated with antioxidants
Resveratrol	200 mg midflight

Gorgeous Girl beware! Although resveratrol is an antioxidant found in red grape skins and red wine, I don't advise imbibing on the flight lest you arrive with a hangover and craggy-looking skin.

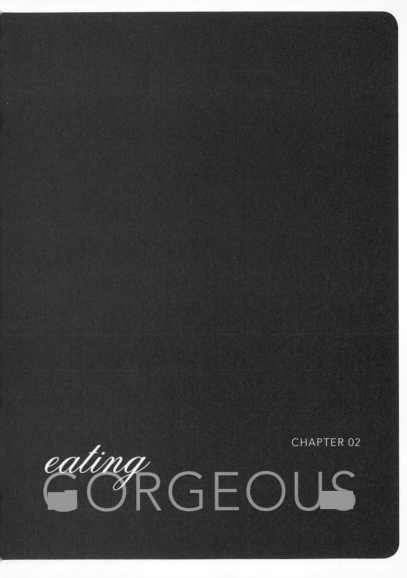

CHAPTER 02

eating
GORGEOUS

THE WHOLE (FOODS) TRUTH

The best foods for us to eat are the ones that are minimally processed—by this I mean foods that don't have additives and aren't heavily packaged, like fresh fruits and veggies, raw nuts and seeds, avocados, whole grains, and proteins. Whole foods are richer in nutrition and contain more vitamins and minerals than their processed counterparts. The body is genetically equipped to break down the foods that it can recognize, as opposed to processed foods, which are much harder to digest and assimilate. Don't worry if you can't eliminate all processed foods; every little thing you do will make a *big* difference.

THE PYRAMID SCHEME

Americans have long considered the Food Guide Pyramid the gold standard for nutritious eating. If that's the case, why is obesity reaching epidemic proportions in North America? As of 2006, the pyramid has a foundation consisting of whole-grain bread, rice, cereal, crackers, and pasta; dark green and orange veggies, beans, and peas are listed next; then fresh, frozen, canned, or dried fruit; milk and dairy come next, followed by a little bit of protein and legumes; and oils are hidden underneath the base. With the exception of brown rice, all the so-called grains listed are processed. There is no differentiation between healthy and unhealthy fats, and no differentiation between sugary dried fruits and low-sugar fresh fruits. Like the pyramid before it, the new pyramid continues to contribute to the fattening of America, since it still advocates a diet based on starches without differentiating between good starches and bad starches. Worse still, most people don't heed the half-cup servings listed. If I were to redo the pyramid, I'd put vegetables and fruits at the base, protein and legumes as the second tier, unprocessed grains as the third tier, healthy fats as the fourth tier, and processed carbs and sugars in the little triangle at the top.

PRIMO PROTEINS

Beef. Make sure your cuts are lean.

Buffalo. Sounds funky, but it's leaner than beef and has more protein. Buffalo also contains healthy amounts of omega-3s.

Chicken and turkey. Both are lean and a great source of protein.

Fish. Wild Alaskan salmon has the lowest mercury content, as do sardines and Alaskan halibut. You can order wild salmon from Vital Choice: www.vitalchoice.com. Canned salmon is also an excellent source of protein. All fish has some mercury, so eat it judiciously. Steer clear of tuna and swordfish, which the EPA warns against due to their high mercury content.

Lamb. A terrific choice for people with a lot of food allergies.

Ostrich. Same as buffalo—give it a whirl! Buffalo and ostrich should be called the "other red meats."

All other game meats. Pheasant, duck, and venison (contains omega-3s) are naturally free-range and rich in nutrition. They're often available at specialty food stores and online.

Whey protein. Though derived from lactose, whey is virtually lactose-free. It is a great way to incorporate protein into your diet and makes a great addition to fruit smoothies, yogurt, and oatmeal.

Whole eggs. Eat both the yolk and the white. The yolk contains more protein than the white, as well as lecithin and choline, which help the liver break down and metabolize cholesterol. Don't believe the hype about eggs raising your cholesterol level; it simply isn't true.

SEXY STARCHES

Barley. This is a whole grain that is rich in fiber and selenium, normalizing your digestion and your blood sugar.

Beans and legumes. These are high in fiber and are released into the bloodstream at a slow, gradual rate. They'll stabilize your blood sugar and control your appetite for hours after you've eaten; they have a minimal impact on your blood sugar.

Brown rice. Loaded with B vitamins, easy to digest, and considered by Eastern medicine to be the most perfectly balanced food, this dietary staple is for you! Make a big pot of it early in the week and reheat portions for dinner.

Other whole grains, such as buckwheat, quinoa, amaranth, and millet. These grains have a small amount of protein and have been around for centuries. If everyone ate these more regularly, we'd all be in great shape!

Corn. Corn is a sugary starch, but it does have health benefits. It is rich in lysine and can help combat cold sores and herpes. Try to buy corn organically whenever possible; a lot of corn is genetically modified and, as a result, has the potential to weaken our immune systems. Please note that corn can be difficult to digest, and you may see it leave your body in the same form it came in. Ewwww!

Fruits. Fruits have fiber and anticancer nutrients and make life sweet. You can buy fresh or frozen ones, but beware of canned fruits and fruit juices, which are high in sugar and less beneficial to your health. Dried fruits are loaded with sugar (even without added sugar), and most people eat too much of them, so buy them sparingly. Think of them as candy. Berries, pears, and apples contain the least sugar, and pineapple, papaya, mangoes, and bananas have the most.

Sweet potatoes. Lower in sugar than white potatoes, sweet potatoes are a superfood that will give you tons of energy. They are chock-full of beta-carotene and potassium and will keep your skin beautiful and improve your immune function.

Vegetables. Dark green leafy vegetables reign as queen of the greens, ranking highest in nutritional content, but any and all vegetables will do your body good! Organic and fresh are best, and organic frozen ones also make a good choice. Fresh vegetable juices are advantageous. Skip the canned veggies, since they are probably devoid of nutrients.

Winter squash. These are sweet and fibrous and will keep you full for hours! They're loaded with beta-carotene, which will help fight colds and flus in the winter.

CHOICES, CHOICES

Q: Is it better to eat a donut that has fewer calories than a bagel but contains more sugar, or a bagel that has more calories but less sugar, or nothing at all for breakfast?

A: How about this: none of the above! I hope by now the message has gotten across that skipping breakfast just ain't an option anymore. Skipping meals raises your cortisol levels so that you feel stressed out and store your calories as fat around your midsection. Not only that, but it can lead you to binge out at your next meal and wreak havoc on your blood sugar. If your choices are limited, try half a bagel with a schmear of cream cheese and some nova (a type of lox); the addition of protein and fat will slow the absorption of sugar into the bloodstream. If you really want a gold star for the day, have some scrambled eggs and slow-cooked oatmeal with berries, a protein smoothie with whey protein, or some Greek yogurt with berries, nuts, and ground flaxseeds. It's chub-free grub that will give you some get-up-and-go-go!

FABULOUS FATS

Contrary to popular belief, the right fats can literally make or break your health.

Coconut oil and fresh coconut fight viruses and boost the immune system, lower cholesterol, help burn body fat, are easy to digest, and are perfect for high-heat cooking.

Grapeseed oil contains omega-6 fats, which do not have the unhealthy ramifications of hydrogenated oils and can withstand high-heat cooking.

About 15 percent of the oils present in **flaxseeds and flaxseed oil** get converted into heart-healthy omega-3s. The seeds are also high in fiber and contain lignans, which help prevent breast and colon cancer and fight constipation. Grind the flaxseeds before eating them and store them in the freezer; store the oil in the refrigerator for optimal freshness.

Olives and olive oil contain omega-9 fats and oleic acid. Oleic acid helps your body absorb the omega-3s found in fish oil and flaxseeds. They sensitize your cells to insulin, helping you to burn fat.

Raw nuts and seeds contain omega-3s and omega-9s. Omega-3s help fight heart disease and keep your cholesterol levels healthy. Raw nuts and seeds also contain trace minerals that stabilize your blood sugar and control your appetite.

SET ME FREE, OMEGA-3S!

Not only do omega-3s spice up your sex life, they also keep your heart thumping and pumping. And, look out drug companies—research proves that omega-3s work even better than statin drugs, without any of the side effects! If you or your loved ones have a history of heart disease, arrhythmias (irregular heartbeat), high blood pressure, elevated heart rate, or clotting, be sure to pack in these lifesaving fats on a daily basis for the rest of your life at a total of 3,000 to 6,000 mg per day. Run this by your doctor first, especially if you are on blood thinners, but for the majority of the population, they're amazing.

margarine: THE FRANKEN-FAT

Why should Gorgeous Girls avoid margarine, hydrogenated and partially hydrogenated vegetable oils, and fried foods? Margarine and fried foods are first-rate drivers in the toxic-fats Grand Prix. Margarine is a man-made substance that is pure poison. Not only does it gum up the insides of your arteries, it also depletes your reserves of good fats. At the molecular level, the structure of margarine is not found in nature, so the body has a very hard time recognizing what it is and therefore can't break it down. What that means for you is a total disruption of your hormone balance and of fatty acids ratios in the body, plus high cholesterol, headaches, joint aches, and a host of other problems related to eating poor-quality fats. (Whereas good fats can help keep all of these symptoms in check.) At the end of the day, I don't care if it's trans fat–free margarine, soy margarine, or bird-turd margarine. If it's a Franken-fat of any form, avoid it! Only the finest, purest, most natural fats will keep you healthy.

FEEL LIKE BUTTAH?
HAVE SOME BUTTAH!

Contrary to popular opinion, butter is natural, safe, and healthy for you to eat. Our bodies need saturated fats to support our bones, protect the liver from toxins, enhance the immune system, and absorb omega-3s. Saturated fats also protect the heart muscle. Scientific evidence does not support the assertion that "artery-clogging" saturated fats cause heart disease. In fact, only 26 percent of the fat in artery clogs is saturated—the rest is unsaturated. So if you want to look and feel like buttah, go ahead and eat some buttah!

DAIRY THERAPY

So pasteurized milk just ain't all it's cracked up to be, as evidenced by all the digestive problems adults face associated with ingesting cows' milk. The culprit isn't the milk—it's the pasteurization process. Once cows' milk is pasteurized, we lose the ability to assimilate its calcium into our bloodstream. Here are some pasteurized milk alternatives:

Raw milk. If you've been dairy-free for years but want to work milk back into your diet, introduce just a few ounces of raw milk per day until your system adjusts. The calcium and nutrients in raw milk are easy to absorb.

Goat milk. Many babes sensitive to cows' milk do just fine on goats' milk. Though a bit pricey, goats' milk is rich in proteins that are much easier to digest than cow's milk.

Almond milk. Unsweetened, enriched almond milk is rich in protein and lower in carbs than other nondairy alternatives. It works well in baking, coffee, tea, or just on the rocks.

Rice milk. This works well in baking, hot beverages, or straight up. Watch out for the sugar content of rice milk, though—it has almost three times the carbs and $1/8$ of the protein of cows' milk.

Avoid soymilk. It contains phytoestrogens that can disrupt hormonal balance and decrease thyroid function.

SAY CHEESE

Cheese is basically a fat with a little bit of protein, so, nutritionally speaking, it should be used in moderation. Hard cheeses can also cause excess mucus production and exacerbate yeast infections because they are naturally high in mold. The best cheeses for you are organic cottage and ricotta, goat, feta, sheep's milk, buffalo milk, and any raw, unpasteurized cheeses you can find. Goat, sheep, and buffalo-milk cheeses are usually better tolerated in people who have allergies or sensitivities to cow's milk. And unpasteurized cheeses are richer in calcium than the more processed brands, since the pasteurization process makes it very difficult for calcium to be absorbed by our bodies.

YOGURT

Yogurt is rich in probiotics, which are the "good" bacteria present in our intestinal tracts. A healthy person normally has about 4 pounds of beneficial bacteria in his or her intestinal tract, and yogurt helps keep that balance intact. Yogurt is low in lactose and very easy to digest, making it no surprise that yogurt has been around for billions of years! Now, here's the catch: To get the most benefit, you must buy the plain kind and sweeten it yourself. A cup of yogurt with the fruit on the bottom has 27 grams of carbs, 26 of which are from sugar. This is far too close to the sugar content in a Snickers bar (my personal favorite), which has 30 grams of sugar. If you thought you were virtuous eating that blueberry yogurt, think twice and make the switch to plain. You can sweeten it with a teaspoon of agave syrup, honey, or maple syrup, as well as fresh fruit, and you'll still have a breakfast or snack that is much lower in sugar. Agave syrup is derived from the nectar of the agave plant. It is naturally low in sugar, but high in flavor; it looks and tastes like honey.

FULL-FAT IS WHERE IT'S AT

Hold on to your hats, ladies—consuming dairy does not have to be a fat-free venture! In fact, consuming fat-free dairy actually does your body a disservice. Fat-free dairy products register in the body as a carbohydrate and can contribute to weight gain as a result. Plus, zero-fat dairy products have far less vitamin D present than their low- or full-fat counterparts. And the taste is just that much better with the presence of rich, smooth, creamy fat particles present. If that doesn't convince you to leave some fat in your dairy, think about this: Studies done on dietary fat intake and breast cancer reveal that it's not the quantity of dietary fat intake that makes a difference in your risk of developing breast cancer, but the quality of the fat. So pick up a tub of your favorite full-fat organic yogurt and bask in the delicious flavor of something that's both delicious and nutritious.

REIGN QUEEN OF GREENS

Incorporating dark green leafy vegetables into your diet will benefit your body in so many ways. Cleaning up your liver, skin, heart, immune system, and intestines are just the beginning of the health and beauty payoffs:

Kale, Brussels sprouts, and broccoli. These veggies help the liver perform the job of detoxification. Broccoli, kale, and Brussels sprouts contain indoles that prevent cancer and glutathione compounds that carry out detoxification reactions.

Barley grass, buckwheat greens, and alfalfa. Barley grass and alfalfa are great sources of protein and contain a wide array of vitamins, minerals, and enzymes that are crucial for maintaining health. Alfalfa contains chlorophyll, which protects against environmental carcinogens. Buckwheat contains rutin and quercetin, two antioxidants that offer cellular protection against oxidative damage; they also protect the body and the liver from alcohol-induced damage. Barley grass is great for treating and healing an upset stomach, diarrhea, gastritis, and inflammatory bowel conditions, all of which can be exacerbated by alcohol.

pest-asides: SHOPPERS' GUIDE

We all know it's best to eat organic. But sometimes organic produce isn't available or is out of our price range. If you have to pick and choose which fruits and veggies to eat organically, refer to the list below to find out which are most contaminated and which are safest. The Environmental Working Group compiled this list. Check out its Web site at www.foodnews.org.

12 Most-Contaminated Fruits and Vegetables (buy these organic)

Apples	Bell Peppers	Celery
Cherries	Imported Grapes	Nectarines
Peaches	Pears	Potatoes
Red Raspberries	Spinach	Strawberries

12 Least-Contaminated Fruits and Vegetables

Asparagus	Avocados	Bananas
Broccoli	Cauliflower	Corn (sweet)
Kiwi	Onions	Mangoes
Papaya	Pineapples	Peas (sweet)

While washing fruits and vegetables will reduce pesticide residues, it can't wash away all of the contamination. Many pesticides are absorbed by the plant and simply can't be removed. Other pesticides are created to adhere to the surface of the produce and stubbornly stick regardless of a good scrub. Peeling rids produce of exterior pesticides, but you lose all of the nutrients in the skin. Your best option is to eat organically as often as you can and always wash your fruits and veggies.

BREAKFASTS OF CHAMPIONS

- Hard-boiled eggs and steel-cut oats with berries. Boil up to 6 eggs at once, and cook steel-cut oats ahead of time in large batches, then reheat single servings for breakfast. Both will keep for one week if refrigerated in an airtight container.

- Protein smoothie: 1 scoop whey protein powder, 2 tablespoons ground flaxseeds, 1 tablespoon natural peanut butter, 1 cup frozen berries or a banana, 1 cup water, and a dash of cinnamon. Blend with ice.

- Plain yogurt with ground flaxseeds, fresh fruit, slivered almonds, and agave or maple syrup

- Vegetable omelet with strawberries

- Smoked salmon with tomato and avocado slices on whole wheat toast

- Whole wheat toast with peanut butter and sliced cantaloupe

SNACK ATTACK

- Hard-boiled eggs

- Celery with peanut butter

- Turkey slices smeared with avocado and rolled up

- Handful of raw nuts

- Apple slices with peanut butter

- Carrots and hummus

- Vegetables and guacamole

- Yogurt and fruit

If the above list is too Pollyanna for you, keep it simple and carry nuts or a piece of fruit with you. No muss, no fuss. Use protein bars for emergency purposes, but don't go overboard, since they usually contain a lot of processed gunk. If you're out of snacks and need to raid the vending machine, stick to pretzels and nuts or cheese and crackers; they're usually the least of the evils. And try to scrounge up some bottled water.

100-CAL GAL

In this supersized culture, we oftentimes eat double the portion size that our bodies actually need. This can lead to an unintentional weight gain of five to ten pounds per year—just enough to guarantee that you won't fit into your threads for too much longer. So what about those 100-calorie snack packs we see everywhere? They do help us to retrain our brains to know what an actual portion size is; this is the same methodology that low-calorie frozen dinners employ. However, these 100-calorie packs are still 100 percent completely processed foods, chock-full of chemicals, sugar, and preservatives. So instead, why not shoot for better options that fall within the 100-calorie range? An apple, ten almonds, two slices of turkey, a hard-boiled egg, or two small squares of dark chocolate all fit the bill and are natural and nutritious.

EATING RIGHT ON DATE NIGHT

Here are some tips on dining out without packing on the pounds. Keep in mind that this info doesn't just apply to date nights. These guidelines work whenever you find yourself in a restaurant:

- Figure out how hungry you are before you start. Rate your hunger on a scale of 1 to 10 whereby a 1 is ravenous and a 10 is overstuffed. Ideally you should start eating at a 2 or 3 and stop somewhere near 5, when you are satisfied.
- If you're worried about eating healthfully but just know you won't be truly satisfied until you have the mac and cheese, order it and commit to stopping when you're full.
- Order a meal that has some protein in it. When your meal arrives, start eating the protein first. Protein is the only nutrient that turns off your body's hunger mechanism and will therefore prevent you from overeating.
- If low-carb eating is your bag, send the bread basket back. Substitute a second vegetable for the starch, and start off with a salad or vegetable-based soup for an appetizer.

Make sure that you get some fat in your meal as well. Fat slows down the absorption of foods in your stomach, making you feel fuller longer.

TO SPLURGE OR NOT TO SPLURGE?

At the end of a tough day, it's completely normal to want to indulge in your favorite comfort foods. Though they may not do a body good, they can satisfy a place within your soul that makes it all worthwhile. The next few pages list real-deal versions of decadent splurges (for those times when nothing else will do) along with their healthier versions so, in a pinch, you can decide whether to splurge or not to splurge.

splurge: ICE CREAM
TO SPLURGE OR NOT TO SPLURGE

A half cup of Ben & Jerry's averages out to 300 calories and 17 grams of fat, depending on the flavor you choose. This means that if you binge on the whole pint, you've just ingested 1,200 calories and 68 grams of fat from ice cream in one sitting! To put this into perspective for you, that's more than a Whopper with cheese, which clocks in at 680 calories and 39 grams of fat.

SOLUTION: SORBET

A half cup of most sorbets checks out at 110 calories, 27 grams of sugar, and 0 grams of fat. Cold comfort, here I come!

splurge: SPAGHETTI
TO SPLURGE OR NOT TO SPLURGE

Most people eat 2 cups of cooked pasta on average, which has 400 calories and a whopping 80 grams of carbohydrates; that's more than twice the amount of carbs found in an 8-ounce glass of regular soda. Yikes! We haven't even taken into account the sauces (tomato sauce has 90 calories per cup; vodka sauce has 380 calories per cup), or the meat (another 200 calories per 3 ounces) and Parmesan cheese (50 calories for 2 tablespoons) that goes on top.

SOLUTION: SOBA NOODLES

Buck up your mood and the nutrient content by switching over to soba noodles, which are made from buckwheat. Two cups of cooked soba noodles contain 220 calories, 48 grams of carbohydrates, and 12 grams of protein. These noodles are delicious tossed with pesto sauce and stir-fried vegetables.

splurge: MAC AND CHEESE
TO SPLURGE OR NOT TO SPLURGE

Loaded with cheese, butter, and whole milk, this pasta dish quickly turns into a diet disaster at 508 calories and 26 grams of fat per serving.

SOLUTION: MAC AND CHEESE MAKEOVER

I found a recipe makeover for a healthier mac and cheese at www.foodfit.com:

> ¾ pound macaroni noodles
> Olive oil for brushing, plus 2 tablespoons
> 2 tablespoons all-purpose flour
> 1½ cups nonfat milk, hot, but not boiling
> ½ cup freshly grated Parmesan cheese
> salt, to taste
> freshly ground black pepper, to taste
> ¼ cup grated sharp cheddar cheese
> ¼ cup bread crumbs

Preheat the oven to 375 degrees F. Cook the macaroni according to package instructions and set aside. Lightly brush a 2-quart casserole dish with olive oil. Bring a large pot of salted water to a boil. In a 2-quart saucepan, whisk the olive oil and flour together over medium heat. Cook until the mixture gives off a "nutty" aroma, about 2 minutes. Slowly whisk in the hot milk and simmer, stirring occasionally, for 5 minutes. Stir in the Parmesan and season with salt and pepper. Set aside. Pour the macaroni into the prepared casserole dish. Pour the milk mixture over it and stir to combine. Sprinkle the grated cheddar over the top, then sprinkle the bread crumbs over the cheese. Bake, uncovered, for about 30 minutes, or until the edges are bubbling and the top is golden brown. Remove from the oven and let stand for 10 minutes before serving. 367 calories per 1½ cup serving.

splurge: MASHED POTATOES
TO SPLURGE OR NOT TO SPLURGE

Considering that a serving of mashed potatoes can have up to 300 calories (gulp!), I had to come up with another option so I could keep my girlish figure—and still enjoy the best of the comfort foods.

SOLUTION: MASHED CAULIFLOWER

Cruciferous cauliflower to the rescue! It's oh-so-healthy and delicious that no one (including you) will know the difference between these guys and whipped potatoes. Take 1 head of cauliflower and chop it up into florets. Throw it in a 2-quart stockpot; add in $1/2$ cup of chicken broth and cover. Steam the cauliflower over medium heat for 20 minutes, or until fork-tender. Add more broth if necessary. Pour the cooked cauliflower and broth into a blender; add $1/4$ cup olive oil and $1/2$ teaspoon sea salt. Blend to desired consistency: less time for a chunkier texture, more for a creamier one. Mmmmmm! 70 calories per 1 cup serving.

splurge: FRENCH FRIES
TO SPLURGE OR NOT TO SPLURGE

A medium McDonald's French fries contains 350 calories and 18 grams of fat. Not the end of the world, but considering that the potatoes fry in cheap, unhealthy oils, there's a lot more danger to eating these than the numbers show. Plus, you're forgetting the Big Mac (560 calories) and the strawberry shake (740 calories) you'll probably order, which brings your meal total up to 1,650 calories.

SOLUTION: BAKED FRIES

Slice up a sweet potato, brush it with coconut oil and sprinkle on some sea salt, and bake it on a cookie sheet in the oven for 45 minutes at 350 degrees F, or until crispy. Or you can buy frozen fries and simply reheat them in the oven. 200 calories per 1 cup serving.

splurge: GOOEY CHOCOLATE BROWNIES
TO SPLURGE OR NOT TO SPLURGE

Two Duncan Hines brownies have 320 calories and 14 grams of fat. Not terrible, but still more than a Snickers bar.

SOLUTION: VEGAN CHOCOLATE CAKE

This recipe takes no more than 10 minutes to make and will keep your hands and mind occupied. You can make two large layers, or bake them in mini loaf pans and freeze one for future cravings.

> 3 cups flour
> 2 cups sugar
> 6 tablespoons cocoa
> 2 teaspoons baking soda
> 1 teaspoon salt
> ¾ cup vegetable oil
> 2 tablespoons vinegar
> 2 teaspoons vanilla
> 2 cups cold water

Mix the dry ingredients together in a large bowl. Add the wet ingredients. Stir until smooth. Bake at 350 degrees F for 30 minutes. Makes two layers of a 9-inch round cake, or one cake baked in a loaf pan. When cool, make a lemon glaze: Combine 2 tablespoons confectioner's sugar with 2 teaspoons lemon juice. Whisk together until well combined and drizzle over cake. 275 calories and 9.6 grams of fat, per 1-inch slice.

splurge: FLUFFERNUTTER SANDWICH
ON WHITE BREAD
TO SPLURGE OR NOT TO SPLURGE

Remember the peanut butter and fluff sandwich? It was the ultimate after-school snack. A Fluffernutter sandwich has 390 calories and creates inner happiness, but it ain't got much in the nutritionally sound department.

SOLUTION:
ALMOND BUTTER WITH ALL-FRUIT PRESERVES ON
WHOLE-GRAIN BREAD

Just a few small changes kicks the nutrient composition up a notch. Almond butter gives you more calcium than peanut butter (2 tablespoons of almond butter has 86 mg; peanut butter has none), as well as 3 grams of fiber and 1 ounce of protein. Both sandwiches have virtually the same amount of calories.

splurge: STORE-BOUGHT HOT CHOCOLATE
TO SPLURGE OR NOT TO SPLURGE

A tall Starbucks hot chocolate with whipped cream has 330 calories, 18 grams of fat, and 28 grams of sugar. Do yourself a favor and make your own, which costs much less and still satisfies your sweet craving.

SOLUTION: HOMEMADE HOT CHOCOLATE

Heat 1 cup of skim milk or water just until it begins to boil. Remove from heat, and stir in 1 tablespoon unsweetened cocoa powder and 2 teaspoons of agave syrup. Stir in some cinnamon and vanilla extract, if you like, for an extra punch, as well as a splash of whole milk. This lower-calorie version has 130 calories if made with milk and 50 calories if made with water. If you like the taste of milk-based hot cocoa but are lactose intolerant, try rice or almond milk, both of which make a delicious cup of hot cocoa.

splurge: GENERAL TSO'S CHINESE CHICKEN

TO SPLURGE OR NOT TO SPLURGE

General Tso's chicken is about the most dangerous chicken dish on the menu—dark meat battered and deep-fried, then cooked with vegetables in a sweet (translation: sugary) and spicy sauce. A 2-cup serving size contains 830 calories, a total of 37 grams of fat, with 7 grams of saturated fat. Yikes!

SOLUTION: SZECHUAN CHICKEN

Szechuan chicken, made with lean white meat and sautéed vegetables, is a far better choice. Two cups contain 500 calories, a total of 21 grams of fat, with 2 grams of saturated fat. If you order steamed brown rice on the side, your fortune cookie will be sure to give you the blessing of health!

splurge: SALT-AND-VINEGAR POTATO CHIPS
TO SPLURGE OR NOT TO SPLURGE

A 1.5-ounce bag has 210 calories, half of which come from fat. And believe you me, it's not from organic olive oil, either. Also bear in mind that the potatoes used to make chips are the supermarket rejects that neither you nor I would bring home for dinner.

SOLUTION: SALTED AIR-POPPED POPCORN

Packed with fiber and low in calories, air-popped popcorn gives you far more bang for your buck: 1 cup has 31 calories, no fat, and 1 gorgeous gram of fiber. So fill up a big bowl and munch to your heart's content—this is a great snack!

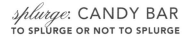

splurge: CANDY BAR
TO SPLURGE OR NOT TO SPLURGE

Standard-sized chocolate bars (like Snickers, Hershey's milk chocolate, and Milky Way) contain roughly 250 calories, mostly from sugars and fat. Treat yourself only once in a blue moon, but don't make it a regular habit!

SOLUTION: DARK CHOCOLATE

Not only does dark chocolate satisfy your sweet tooth, but you'll get the benefits of antioxidants, too. Plus, you may feel extra love when you eat chocolate. Phenylethylamine is a compound that naturally occurs in chocolate. When consumed, it releases endorphins in your brain, which produce a mild feeling of euphoria, mimicking the sensation of being in love. Other compounds naturally occurring in chocolate include scrotonin, theobromine, and anandamide, which all elevate mood, increase circulation, and enhance sensory perception. One ounce of dark chocolate (70 percent cocoa content or higher) contains about 154 calories, 12 grams of fat, 2 grams of fiber, and 2 grams of protein. Spread a little natural peanut butter on your chocolate if you'd like a homemade mini peanut butter cup!

RAH, RAH, RAW!

What exactly does it mean to go raw? Eating raw ensures that foods remain rich in enzymes and nutrients with only minimal heating to keep those natural enzymes present intact. All the foods on a raw diet are uncooked, virtually unheated, unprocessed, and, ideally, organic. The foods, therefore, are naturally plant-based: uncooked fruits and vegetables, nuts, seeds, sprouted grains, cold-pressed olive oil, and certain spices and seasonings.

If you feel like you've tried everything to get your health on track and nothing else has worked, this may very well make you feel better. Because the raw foods diet is alkaline, it can help reestablish the biochemical balance in your body. So, if you are prone to symptoms from arthritis, gas and bloating, constipation, sinusitis, and yeast infections, or if you just want to give your body a much-needed change, the raw foods diet is worth considering. In my professional experience, however, you most probably won't need to go to this extreme to see results in your body, but it's also good to know that the option is available. If going raw seems too extreme for you, consider adding more raw foods and vegetable juices into your diet. You'll still enjoy greater balance and will see positive changes in your health.

THE USUAL SUSPECTS

It's worth mentioning what we nutritional peeps like to call The Sensitive Seven—foodstuffs that antagonize the immune system. I have treated countless patients who were given diagnoses of colitis, eczema, dermatitis, arthritis, and any other *itis* you can come up with, but get this: 99 percent of their illnesses cleared up with dietary changes alone. So, if you're sick of being sick, or just want to give yourself 24-carat health, try removing these foods from your diet: wheat, dairy, sugar, peanuts, eggs, corn, and soy. These foods are implicated in numerous crimes against your poor intestinal tract and should be sentenced to at least six months in the pokey before getting out for parole! This elimination diet is cost-effective and will likely save you thousands of dollars in doctors visits, medication, and time spent in the waiting room.

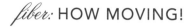

fiber: HOW MOVING!

Fiber regulates your bowel movements and purifies your system.

- Fiber acts as an internal detoxifying agent and helps remove pesticides and toxins.
- Fiber is a prebiotic and builds up the good bacteria in the gut and digestive enzymes.
- Fiber helps you feel fuller longer and controls your appetite and encourages fat-burning.

If you eat pounds of fiber daily and are still constipated, make sure you up your daily water intake. If you up your fiber intake without upping your water intake you're asking for trouble! And if you're contemplating fiber supplements, skip the over-the-counter junk. Instead, add 1 to 2 tablespoons of ground flaxseed to your oatmeal or yogurt each morning; I guarantee you the Earth will start moving!

SH*T HAPPENS

Trying to get more fiber into your diet but not sure how? Before you go out looking for Super Colon Blow cereal, there are a few things you should know about fiber. Fiber is found not only in cereals and bran. Oh no, my dear. Your friend fiber is found in all types of foods.

There are two types of fiber: soluble and insoluble. Soluble fiber abounds in beans and legumes, oats, barley, rye, plums, berries, broccoli, carrots, sweet potatoes, onions, and psyllium seed husks. Insoluble fiber is in the skins of fruits and vegetables. You need both types of fiber, so eat a wide range of fruits and veggies. One of my favorite forms of fiber is ground flaxseeds, which contains 8 grams of insoluble fiber per 2 tablespoons and is a known preventative to breast and colon cancer.

AS THE STOMACH CHURNS

If you picked up more than just your salad at lunch and are now grappling with Montezuma's revenge or have already tossed your cookies, try one of the following remedies and always keep them on hand when you travel. If you've dined at a suspicious restaurant, employ these treatments as a precaution, otherwise you may be the star in your very own dramedy, *As the Stomach Churns.* . . .

- **Probiotics:** Take 1 capsule (aim for 8 billion organisms per capsule) every hour until diarrhea stops; then take 8–16 billion per day to keep your digestive tract healthy. If you are vomiting, wait until vomiting resolves, then take 1 capsule every 6 hours for 24 hours; then 3 capsules per day for 2 days; then 1 capsule per day for maintenance as a long-term preventative for food poisoning.
- **Oil of oregano:** Take 1 drop in a glass of water or tomato juice 3 times daily for diarrhea or suspected food-borne illnesses. You'll smell like a pizza, but that's better than feeling icky for longer than you need to.
- **For severe diarrhea:** Try to stay as hydrated as you can with diluted apple juice, water, and chamomile tea. Drink ginger tea to soothe a nauseated tummy, as well as peppermint tea. Munching on ice chips is another soothing way to get some fluids in.

THERE ARE OTHER FISH IN THE SEA . . .

We all need to lube our internal combustion engines. With so many different types of oils out there, how do you know which one is appropriate for you? And is one better than the others? You bet your omega-3s there is!

- **Krill oil** has more antioxidants than regular fish oil and carries omega-3s in the form of phospholipids, making them much easier to absorb. Krill oil won't cause any unpleasant belching, and it gets your serotonin levels up up up! Taking krill oil is also good for the environment, as the ocean's supply is incredibly abundant; this is not true of all other fish in the sea. Take 4 capsules daily for general wellness.
- **Cod-liver oil** is fantabulous in the winter months because it contains the immune-boosting vitamins A and D. This means a better chance at beating respiratory infections, colds and flus, seasonal affective disorder, and bone loss. Take 1 teaspoon per 50 pounds of body weight daily.
- **Wild sockeye salmon oil** is rich in omega-3s, vitamin D, and astaxanthin, so you can't go too wrong here, either. But make sure you get it from Alaska, which is the only state to make fish farming illegal. This ensures you get a squeaky-clean product free of mercury and PCBs, with all the essential oils still intact. Take 4 capsules daily for overall wellness.

Note to Gorgeous Self: All supplements should be taken with food.

EVERY GIRL LOVES FRESH FLOURS

Baking can be a snap, even if you want to take it up a notch with über-healthy substitutions for flour products. Almond flour is an excellent substitute for any flour and can be used to coat meat, bake cakes, and make crusts. It's a bit pricier, but it's a superdelish and healthy way to add more fiber and trace minerals to recipes while cutting out gluten and processed foods.

You can also get adventurous in the kitchen with coconut flour, which has more fiber and protein than white flour. The texture is fine and powdery and can be used in all types of baking, smoothies, and even as a bread-crumb substitute. The beauty of coconut flour is that the saturated fat is incredibly stable in high heat conditions and kills off viruses and harmful bacteria that can weaken our immune systems. So if you think healthy baking is an oxymoron, think again!

CHOCOLATE CAKE

½ cup butter or coconut oil
¼ cup cocoa powder
¼ cup coconut milk, rice milk, or almond milk
9 eggs
1 cup, plus 2 tablespoons agave syrup
¾ teaspoon salt
1 teaspoon vanilla
¾ cup sifted coconut flour
¾ teaspoon baking powder

Preheat the oven to 350 degrees F. Melt the butter in a saucepan over medium heat. Add the cocoa powder and coconut milk and mix well. Remove from heat and set aside. In a large mixing bowl, whisk together the eggs, agave syrup, salt, and vanilla. Stir in the cocoa mixture. Combine the coconut flour and baking powder, then whisk into the batter until there are no lumps. Pour the batter into a greased 8-by-8-by-2- or 9-by-9-by-2-inch pan. Bake for 35 minutes or until a knife inserted into center comes out clean. Cool, then cover with frosting.

Frosting
¾ cups organic whipping cream
2 tablespoons agave syrup
2 tablespoons unsalted butter
¼ pound milk chocolate, chopped
¼ pound dark chocolate (60 percent cocoa content), chopped

Combine the cream, syrup, and butter in a large heavy saucepan. Whisk over medium heat until the mixture begins to simmer. Add the chopped chocolates. Reduce heat to low and whisk until the frosting is smooth, about 1 minute. Transfer to large bowl.

Fill another large bowl with ice. Set the bottom of bowl with frosting atop the ice bath. Whisk the frosting until it's cool and begins to thicken, about 8 minutes. Place frosting bowl on your work surface.

Using an electric mixer, beat the frosting until its color lightens and the frosting becomes thick enough to hold soft peaks, about 2 minutes (the frosting will continue to thicken the longer it stands).

Place cake flat side up on an 8-inch cardboard round. Top with the frosting, spreading over the top and sides of the cake (if the frosting becomes stiff, stir gently with a spatula to loosen).

ALMOND-FLOUR MUFFINS

¾ cup unsalted butter
¾ cup agave syrup
4 eggs
½ cup almond or rice milk
1 teaspoon vanilla
1½ cups almond flour
½ cup organic coconut flour
2 teaspoons baking powder
¼ teaspoon sea salt

Preheat the oven to 350 degrees F. Using an electric hand mixer, cream together butter and syrup until smooth. Add in the eggs, one at a time, and beat until fully blended. Add the milk and vanilla and mix until combined. In a separate bowl, combine the flours, salt, and baking powder. Beat the dry ingredients into the wet ingredients with the mixer. Beat until creamy. Fill a buttered muffin pan until the cups are ¾ full and bake for 15 to 20 minutes. Serve with fresh fruit and whipped cream.

SEXY SUBSTITUTES

For some healthy alternatives that do a bang-up job in the kitchen, try the following substitutes. You'll still be able to look yourself in the mirror in the morning when you cook with these savory treats because they'll do your body good. Talk about having your cake and eating it, too!

INSTEAD OF . . .	TRY . . .
Corn syrup	Agave syrup
White flour	Almond flour or coconut flour
Milk chocolate	Dark chocolate
Cow's milk	Almond milk or rice milk
Shortening	Butter
Vegetable oil	Grapeseed oil

ginger: THE ORIGINAL SPICE GIRL

When it comes to health, nothing beats ginger for soothing coughs and congestion. Sadly, it's sorely underutilized in foods today; we often see pickled ginger on the side of a sushi plate or candied ginger in fancy restaurants, but it's hard to find in many other foods. Ginger warms you from the inside out and has a zesty punch that will penetrate even the stuffiest of noses. For some homemade herbal goodness, try this recipe for ginger tea: Peel and slice up an entire fresh ginger root (about 1-2 ounces) and drop it into a 2-quart saucepan filled with water. Boil for 10 minutes, pour into your favorite mug, and drink it throughout the day for blessed relief.

turmeric: YELLOW GOLD

Turmeric is a bright yellow spice rich in manganese, iron, and B_6. It is native to Indonesia and southern India, making it the base for curries and other flavorful dishes.

Multiple studies have shown turmeric's benefits in acting as a natural anti-inflammatory and antioxidant, preserving our precious brain cells and warding off Alzheimer's disease, fighting prostate cancer, heart disease, rheumatoid arthritis, inflammatory bowel disease, and colon cancer.

The yellow pigment of turmeric is curcumin, which is the primary pharmacological agent in turmeric. It works hard for the money! In numerous studies, the pharmacological benefits of curcumin have been shown to be comparable to steroids (like cortisone) and NSAIDS (nonsteroidal anti-inflammatory drugs) (like Motrin), but without the toxic side effects (ulcers, intestinal bleeding, decreased white blood cell count). Nutrients are nutrients and drugs are drugs, but in this case, I do believe we can all be friends!

For fare with flair, add turmeric to egg salad, lentils, salad dressings, cauliflower, and mayonnaise. Handle this herb with care; wear gloves and avoid getting it on your clothing, unless you like bright yellow stains all over your hands and threads.

GOJI BERRIES FOR YOUR TWIGS AND BERRIES

If I had my druthers, I'd call these little suckers go-go berries—they pack quite an energy punch! Goji berries are mostly found in their dried form and look similar to red raisins. In traditional Chinese medicine, they are used to enhance immune-system function, improve eyesight, protect the liver, boost sperm production, improve circulation, and promote longevity. Goji berries are a rich source of zeaxanthin, a carotenoid beneficial for retinal health, and vitamin C.

To punch up your morning oatmeal or yogurt, rehydrate the goji berries by soaking them in water for 10 minutes before adding them to your breakfast. Or, just drop them raw into your trail mix as a snack. And to ignite your mojo, be sure to enjoy them every day.

Note: Goji berries are indigenous to China and are often heavily treated with pesticides. So be sure to purchase only the organically grown.

CAULIFLOWER POWER

Cauliflower and other cruciferous veggies are dazzlingly high in glucosinolates—cancer-fighting chemicals that get broken down in the digestive tract to isothiocynates and indole-3-carbinol. These all help regulate the body's detoxification enzymes and ultimately eliminate cancer-causing substances. Look out, colon cancer! Beware, breast and prostate cancers! Cauliflower is also a rich source of selenium—an almighty trace mineral that strengthens the immune system and wards off cancer.

Convenience factor: Cauliflower will keep in the fridge for five to seven days, but if you buy precut cauliflower, it will only keep for two days. Is the tradeoff worth it? You decide . . .

Check out page 62 for a cauliflower recipe that's a great substitute for high-calorie mashed potatoes. You won't be able to tell the difference!

broccoli: THE CELLULAR MAKEOVER

I bet you've never thought of broccoli as a fashion-forward vegetable, have you? Broccoli contains high levels of glucoraphanin, which stimulates enzymes that cleanse our cells, detoxify carcinogens, and suppress the growth of cancerous tumors. It's sort of a closet consultant of sorts—someone who cleans out your internal closet and gets rid of your culottes and Day-Glo neon Lycra outfits circa 1980! The good news is that you really don't have to eat gobs of the little green trees to benefit: Just a half cup cooked is an ample source of more than 1,000 IU of vitamin A, as well as vitamin C (an orange's worth), calcium (as much as 4 ounces of milk), iron, folic acid, and potassium.

And it's true what they say about the darker the berry, the sweeter the juice; the blue-green florets contain more beta-carotene and vitamin C than their lighter-colored counterparts.

To smack the nutritional value out of the park, steam broccoli and drizzle it with olive oil, lemon juice, and fresh garlic. Or steam it, blanch it in ice water, and toss the florets with soba noodles and wild Alaskan salmon.

chocolate: NAUGHTY AND NICE

An ounce of naughty can feel great. And an ounce of dark chocolate every day can improve insulin resistance and sensitivity while lowering systolic blood pressure and the risk of blood clotting. But, here's the catch, it has to be processed properly and have only the highest quality ingredients. To ensure you're eating good-quality dark chocolate, make sure the ingredient list includes only these fab five: chocolate liquor, cocoa butter, sugar, vanilla, and lecithin. Most cocoa is processed in ways that destroy the majority of the beneficial polyphenolic bioflavanoids, so by going for pure, organic, simple ingredients, you'll ensure that you can have your chocolate and eat it, too.

Don't like dark chocolate, you say? I'm afraid that milk chocolate isn't a good substitute. Dairy interferes with the antioxidants found in dark chocolate, so milk chocolate doesn't have the same health benefits of dark, and white chocolate technically isn't chocolate. If you're a die-hard milk-chocolate lover, try to wean yourself off. Buy dark chocolate varieties with nuts or dried fruit to make it more palatable. You can go green with chocolate, too—look for bars made with ethically traded cacao beans that support sustainable forest farmland and their species.

And remember, a little dab will do ya—break off just an ounce a day for healthful benefits.

DON'T GO DOWN WITH THE SHIP!

Congratulations! After months of speed-dating, being wingman for your best friend, and toning those gorgeous abs, you've done it—you've scored yourself a relationship! The good news is that you're being wined and dined, and your skin is aglow from all the delicious lovin' you're getting. The bad news is that you're spending more time in bed than at the gym, the romantic dinners are wreaking havoc on your waistline, and all the extra booze with dinner is wiping out your resolve. Over time, you got really comfy with your man and yourself, and you let your good intentions slip. It's so much easier to stay in and order Chinese than muster up the energy to cook something healthy, right?

But before you let it all go downhill, remind yourself what all that hard work was about in the first place: a commitment you made to *yourself* to look and feel great. You loved and cared for yourself when you were single, and that side of you needs to stay alive and present while you're in a relationship. So, rather than go against the grain, think of ways to incorporate your original drive into your couples routine. Couples that cook romantic dinners and go to the gym together stay together!

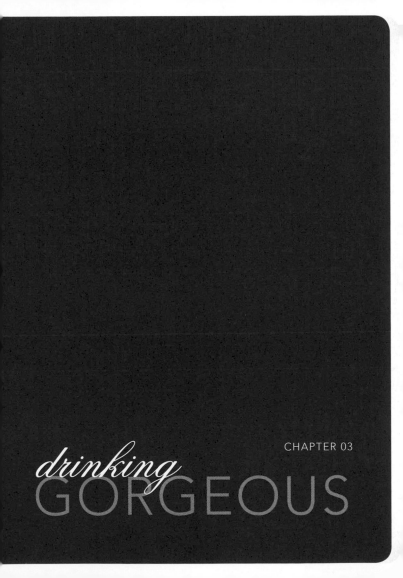

CHAPTER 03

drinking
GORGEOUS

water: LIQUEFIED AND LOVING IT!

To calculate exactly how many ounces of water you need a day, divide your body weight in half; that's the number of ounces to shoot for. So a 150-pound person would need to drink 75 ounces of water, or roughly nine glasses (8 ounces per glass) of water per day. For every 20 minutes you exercise, you will need to drink an additional 4 to 8 ounces of water. For every caffeinated or alcoholic beverage you consume, you will need to drink another 8 ounces of water to compensate for their dehydrating effects.

What drinks are the best antidotes for dehydration? The best and most pure is, of course, filtered water. So make your way over to the watercooler, pronto! If you're not crazy about plain old water, you've got other options. Grab a bottle of seltzer, dilute a shot of pomegranate juice into a glass of water, or chill out with herbal teas. Spice up regular water with slices of lemons, limes, oranges, or cucumbers for a delicious and healthy treat! And don't forget to invest in a good at-home filter to remove impurities such as lead, rust, chlorine, and cryptosporidia from the tap water.

BOOZE NEWS

Here's a handy breakdown of calories in different types of drinks:

Beer. Nonalcoholic and alcoholic beer actually have the same number of calories: 148 calories in a 12-ounce serving. Light beer has around 99 calories per 12 ounces.

Wine. Dry wine contains fewer calories than sweeter wine. A glass of dry wine, including Champagne, has about 106 calories and a glass of sweet dessert wine a whopping 226.

Hard alcohol. The calories in gin, rum, vodka, and whiskey depend on the proof, which is twice the percentage of alcohol. It's easy to guess which has more calories: The higher the proof, the higher the calories. Here's the damage:
- Double shot of 80-proof liquor—97 calories
- Double shot of 90-proof liquor—110 calories
- Double shot of 100-proof liquor—124 calories

Liqueurs. The calorie content of other types of liquor varies greatly. Watch the really sweet stuff. A serving of schnapps has 108 calories, and crème de menthe will set you back 186 calories.

Mixed drinks. Obviously, the larger the mixed drink, the higher the calorie content. Check out the sidebar, Where Do Your Drinks Weigh In?, on page 92 for more details.

WHERE DO YOUR DRINKS WEIGH IN?

Unless otherwise noted, the calories listed for wine and cocktails are based on a 4-ounce serving, and beer servings are 12 ounces.

Chardonnay:	90 calories
Kahlúa and cream:	90 calories (1.5 ounces)
Red wine:	90 calories
Michelob Ultra:	95 calories
Coors Light beer:	102 calories
Champagne, dry:	106 calories
Gimlet:	110 calories
Miller Light beer:	110 calories
Schlitz Light beer:	110 calories
Sangria:	115 calories
Bloody Mary:	115 calories
Amstel Light beer:	120 calories
Whiskey sour:	122 calories
Jack Daniel's and Coke:	129 calories
Rum and Diet Coke:	133 calories
Mimosa:	137 calories
Samuel Adams:	145 calories
Miller Genuine Draft:	148 calories
Hot toddy:	150 calories (3 ounces)
Newcastle Brown Ale:	150 calories

Strawberry daiquiri: 150 calories

Mudslide: 155 calories

Irish coffee: 159 calories

Budweiser: 160 calories

Dos Equis: 160 calories

Heineken beer: 160 calories

Samuel Adams Boston Lager: 160 calories

Gin and tonic: 171 calories

Pete's Wicked Ale: 174 calories

Cosmopolitan: 179 calories

Manhattan: 183 calories

Chocolate martini: 188 calories

Guinness Extra Stout: 190 calories

Screwdriver: 208 calories

Red Bull with vodka: 210 calories

Strawberry margarita: 210 calories

Martini: 210 calories

Rum and Coke: 240 calories

Frozen margarita: 246 calories

Eggnog: 305 calories

Mai tai: 306 calories

Piña colada: 342 calories

GATORADE GALS

You may wonder how the world ever survived before Gatorade existed. Sports drinks are designed to replace electrolytes lost during exercise, such as sugar, salt, and other trace minerals. Newer sports drinks on the market also include amino acids to help the body recover more quickly from strenuous exercise. Energy drinks simply contain boatloads of caffeine and sugar, and although they'll put some pep in your step, they are not designed to improve your workout performance. All of these drinks contain plenty of Day-Glo artificial dyes, as well as calories and sugar. And the sports drinks often use sweeteners in the form of fructose, which can cause a hypoglycemic response if consumed too far ahead of the event itself. My recommendation: Only use sports drinks when participating in an endurance exercise event lasting longer than ninety minutes (sex does not count here, sorry), and feel free to dilute those sports drinks by 50 percent or make your own concoction. Even better, for a caffeine buzz that also has antioxidants, brew yourself some fresh tea and call it a day!

NUTRITIOUS AND DELICIOUS: COCKTAIL MAKEOVERS

In today's health-conscious age, we all want to do just a little better for ourselves without going completely overboard. By giving your cocktails a makeover you are doing something healthy for yourself. Small changes make a big difference!

INSTEAD OF . . .	TRY . . .
Apple martini	Green tea martini
Cosmopolitan	Pomegranate martini
Vodka on the rocks	Citron vodka with raspberry club soda
Red Bull with vodka	Diet Vanilla Coke with vanilla vodka
Gin martini	Gimlet
Gin and tonic	Gin and Diet Sprite
Dark ale	Light beer

SHAKEN OR STIRRED?

Note to Gorgeous Self: If you're making a martini or any drink you're going to be serving in a martini glass, it is imperative that you chill the glasses beforehand; this will keep the drink cold and remarkably smooth when it is served. Here are my tips for a no-fail martini: Fill the martini glasses with ice and water and set them in the freezer for two minutes while you're mixing the drinks. When you're ready to pour the mixed drink, pull the glasses out from the freezer and pour out the ice water. Your glasses will be chilled and ready to go! Also make sure you prep the bar area ahead of time: slice up lemons and limes, fill the ice bucket, and keep toothpicks skewered with fat, juicy green cocktail olives in a highball glass so they can be plucked out and dunked right into your drink. Voilà!

COCKTAIL MAKEOVERS

Vodka Martini
1½ ounces vodka
½ teaspoon dry vermouth
3 cocktail olives

Pour the vodka into a shaker that is halfway filled with ice. Shake vigorously for 20 seconds. Set aside. Pour the dry vermouth into a martini glass. Swish the vermouth around the glass and shake the remnants out. Pour in the ice-cold vodka and add in the olives. If you like your martinis dirty, add in a splash of olive juice.

Bonus: Olives are chock-full of essential fatty acids to help your liver metabolize it all.

Pomegranate Cosmos
¾ cup vodka
⅓ cup triple sec
⅓ cup fresh lime juice
⅓ cup pomegranate juice

Fill a pitcher with ice. Add vodka, triple sec, fresh lime juice, and pomegranate juice. Stir until well combined and thoroughly chilled. *Makes 4 cosmos.*

Bonus: Pomegranate juice is chock-full of antioxidants, providing some protection for your cells while you drink.

Green Tea-Tini

1 ounce green tea, chilled
2 ounces Grey Goose citron vodka
¼ ounce Grand Marnier
1 teaspoon fresh lime juice

Pour the green tea, vodka, and Grand Marnier into a shaker that is halfway filled with ice. Shake vigorously for 20 seconds. Set aside. Pour the lime juice into a martini glass. Swish the lime juice around the glass and shake the remnants out into the sink. Pour the shaker ingredients into a martini glass and garnish with lime slices.

Bonus: Green tea is also loaded with polyphenols and antioxidants, improving the nutritional content of your alcoholic bevvie.

Gin and Sin

1½ ounces gin
1½ ounces freshly squeezed orange juice
1 ounce freshly squeezed lemon juice
2 dashes grenadine

Put all ingredients in a shaker that is halfway filled with ice. Shake vigorously for 20 seconds and strain into a chilled martini glass.

Bonus: The freshly squeezed lemon juice will support liver function and detoxification.

MOCKTAILS

Pomegranate Mimosa
1 glass sparkling cider
½ ounce pomegranate juice
Lemon peel for garnish

Pour sparkling cider into a champagne flute. Add the pomegranate juice. Use the lemon peel as a garnish that you can drop right into the mimosa.

Bonus: This is a far more nutritious drink than soda, and it is much prettier to look at!

Baby Bellini
2 ounces peach nectar
1 ounce fresh lemon juice
Chilled sparkling cider

Pour the peach nectar and the lemon juice into a chilled champagne flute. Stir well. Add cider to fill the remainder of the glass. Stir again gently

Bonus: This also offers more benefits than soda and can be used as a virgin drink between alcoholic courses.

BEER BEFORE LIQUOR . . .

Is the saying "Beer before liquor, never sicker; liquor before beer, never fear" physiologically accurate? No, my darlings. I'm afraid it's not that simple. Rather, it's mixing different types of alcohol that's generally a bad idea. It's possible that the reasoning behind the proverb is that it's easier on your body to absorb weaker alcoholic drinks, like beer, later in the evening. But any piece of advice regarding alcohol consumption that contains the line "never fear" is obviously pretty suspect.

GORGEOUS UNDER THE INFLUENCE

In general, hangovers are more common with distilled, stronger alcoholic drinks and less so with wines and beer. You're a lot less likely to get hangovers if you follow a few simple rules:

- Skip the sugary daiquiris, margaritas, and cosmopolitans.
- To avoid getting too tipsy too quickly, order water or club soda with lime between cocktails.
- Skip the mixers. I'm not saying slam down shots, but sipping whiskey or vodka means you'll avoid a whole lot of sugar. Flavored club soda will make most drinks pretty palatable.
- Say no to caffeine. Caffeine suppresses ADH (antidiuretic hormone), which makes you pee more, ultimately dehydrating you.
- Finish drinking early enough to let your body metabolize as much alcohol as possible before going to bed.
- Try to get enough rest to enable your body to burn off the alcohol. Generally you burn off about two-thirds of a drink per hour; this rate may slow down while you're sleeping.
- If you take a painkiller to offset a potential headache, skip the acetaminophen (found in Tylenol) and take something ibuprofen-based (like Advil).

SHORT-TERM MEASURES FOR CURTAILING THOSE POST-PARTY HANGOVERS

Key tips to offset a hangover:

- Bar snacks are there for a reason. Grab some finger foods while you imbibe.
- There are no hard-and-fast rules as to whether a protein-rich meal like steak or a carb-based meal will better prevent you from absorbing alcohol too quickly.
- Avoid too many salty snacks while drinking. The sodium content of these foods makes you thirstier, and you will end up refilling your glass faster.
- Never mix your alcohols. Be scientific about it; don't even switch from red wine to white wine or pinot blanc to pinot grigio at the same sitting. The same rules apply to hard alcohols; stick to one brand as much as possible.
- Remember to pace yourself during the night. Alternate naughty alcoholic drinks with angelic virgin versions, or even just plain water.
- If you don't usually smoke but you dabble while drinking, look out! This will intensify your hangover the next day.
- Splurge on top-shelf liquors when drinking, even in mixed drinks. The cheaper versions are less processed and filtered than the expensive versions and can leave you with an unwanted headache even early in the evening.

HALT THE HANGOVER

If you know you're going to be out for a few drinks, but don't want to suffer from a hangover the next day, consider taking cysteine (200 mg) plus vitamin C (600 mg) prior to drinking, with each drink, and once again right after you finish drinking. Many drinkers find that this strategy results in a hangover-free following day. (All the extra water you must drink when taking these pills certainly doesn't hurt, either!)

- Some people replace regular cysteine in this combination with N-acetyl cysteine (NAC), although this form may be slightly less effective.
- The addition of vitamin B_6 (50 mg) to this regime further enhances its effectiveness for preventing hangovers.
- Also take 150 mg of milk thistle twice per day, with 250 mg of schisandra.
- Take 2 capsules of evening primrose oil (1,000 mg each) before heading out on the town.
- DMAE has also been shown to help prevent hangovers: Take 200 mg per day.

AFTER A NIGHT ON THE TOWN, TRY THIS

- When you get home after a night of drinking, drink plenty of water before you go to bed. This will prevent the dehydration that accompanies most hangovers. A little Gatorade can also help replace lost electrolytes, though it's not ideal because it contains high-fructose corn syrup, which is a cheaply processed, poor-quality sweetener.
- Take 150 mg of milk thistle and 250 mg of schisandra. Before you go out, put them in the bathroom next to a big glass of water, so when you get home you won't forget.
- Take 1,000 mg of N-acetyl cysteine and 500 mg of vitamin C.
- Take two 1,000 mg capsules of evening primrose oil, too.

THE MORNING AFTER, TRY THIS

- Take 400 mg of magnesium.
- Take 1,000 mg of N-acetyl cysteine.
- Take 1,500–6,000 mg of MSM.
- For a sour stomach, take a heaping teaspoon of glutamine powder mixed in water.
- For headaches, take 800 mg of willow bark. Willow bark contains salicin, a substance used in aspirin.
- Nux vomica will help relieve gas, bloating, and a sour stomach. Take the 6c potency in 4 drops or pellets every hour.
- Drink tomato juice. It contains fructose, a type of sugar that helps your body metabolize alcohol more quickly.
- Eat crackers and honey. Honey has a high level of fructose.
- Refresh your sour palate with peppermint. Take it in tea form or by chewing the leaves. Peppermint is a carminative, a substance that removes accumulated gas from the stomach and intestines to relax your intestines. Make the tea by pouring 1 cup of boiling water over 1 to 2 teaspoons of the dried herb; cover; steep for 15 minutes; strain. Drink 1 or 2 cups as soon as you can.

vitamins: RESCUE REMEDIES AND HANGOVER HELPERS

Evening primrose oil. An essential fatty acid that improves circulation, helps regulate inflammation, and relieves pain. The main active ingredient of evening primrose oil is gamma-linoleic acid (GLA), an omega-6 fatty acid that can also be found in borage and black currant oils. *Dosage:* 1,000–2,000 mg per day.

NAC (N-acetyl cysteine). An altered form of the amino acid cysteine, commonly found in food. NAC helps the body synthesize glutathione, an important antioxidant. In animals, the antioxidant activity of NAC protects the liver from the adverse effects of exposure to several toxic chemicals. In humans, NAC helps drive out toxins acquired from booze and tobacco smoke. *Dosage:* 1,000–1,500 mg per day.

Vitamin B_6 and lipoic acid. Vitamin B_6 and lipoic acid are key sulfur-containing nutrients that may be depleted by alcohol and may help with acetaldehyde detoxification. Vitamin B_6 has been proven to further enhance the ability of the combination of cysteine plus vitamin C to prevent hangovers. *Dosage:* 300 mg per day of B_6; 300 mg per day of lipoic acid.

Vitamins C and E. Research shows that vitamins C and E and the amino acid cysteine act as an antioxidant force to counter acetaldehyde-produced free radicals, helping to protect against long-term damage. *Dosage:* 500–1,000 mg per day of vitamin C; 400 IU of vitamin E—try to find a food-based supplement for these.

Magnesium. Many of the symptoms of hangovers are believed to come from the magnesium depletion that occurs when you drink alcohol. Supplementing your diet with additional magnesium helps counteract hangover symptoms that stem from a lack of magnesium. *Dosage*: 400 mg per day of magnesium glycinate (a highly absorbable form of magnesium).

DMAE. A clinical study found that when dimethylaminoethanol (DMAE), a derivative of choline, was taken for at least six weeks, it resulted in subjects being free of the headaches and irritability that normally occur with hangovers. *Dosage*: 200 mg per day.

MSM. Methylsulfonylmethane (MSM) is a good source of sulfur, which may counteract the ability of acetaldehyde to initiate hangovers. This therapy has not yet been tested in clinical trials, but many of my "research subjects" claim that it rapidly (within 20 minutes) alleviates the symptoms of hangovers. *Dosage*: 1,000–3,000 mg per day.

Zinc. The enzyme acetaldehyde dehydrogenase stimulates the conversion of hangover-causing acetaldehyde (derived from alcoholic drinks) into acetic acid (used for energy production). Plenty of zinc should theoretically maximize the availability of this enzyme to divert acetaldehyde toward energy production rather than permitting acetaldehyde to exert its toxic effects, causing hangovers. *Dosage*: 25–50 mg per day.

Silymarin (milk thistle). Milk thistle is a potent antioxidant that has been shown to protect the liver and enhance its functioning. It prevents the depletion of glutathione, a substance crucial in the liver's detoxification role. It also helps promote the regeneration of new liver cells. Alcohol depletes glutathione, but because of its antioxidant properties, milk thistle helps replenish glutathione. Glutathione is a cofactor for antioxidant enzymes and helps recycle other antioxidants, like vitamins C and E. *Dosage*: 400 mg per day.

Schisandra. Studies with animals suggest that schisandra may protect the liver from toxic damage, improve liver function, and stimulate cell regrowth in the liver. Schisandra seeds contain more than a dozen liver-protective compounds. It appears that schisandra lignans protect the liver by activating the enzymes in liver cells that produce glutathione, the liver's most important antioxidant. *Dosage*: 250 mg per day, either in tablet or liquid tincture form.

HAIR OF THE DOG?

Although the phrase "the hair of the dog that bit you" originally referred quite literally to a cure for dog bites, people often use the phrase when having an "eye-opener" the morning after a big night out drinking. Why? you ask. To try to alleviate the symptoms of a hangover by drinking more alcohol! If you're looking for a convenient excuse to crack open a can of Schlitz at 10 A.M. on a Sunday, then go for it. But as your Venus de No-No, I must warn you that it's not such a great idea, since your body has not yet finished metabolizing all the alcohol from the night before. Let's take a quick look at some of the supposed morning-after "remedies," just for fun:

- Bloody Mary
- Mimosa
- Black Velvet (a mix of champagne and flat Guinness)
- Tomato juice and beer (Hemingway's tonic)
- A "red-eye": whiskey, coffee, Tabasco sauce, a raw egg, pepper, and orange juice blended together
- Raw eggs
- Hot coffee
- Lots of ice-cold Coke, ginger ale, or Gatorade
- A greasy breakfast

The Greeks are my heroes: They munched on cabbage! Fantastic liver support.

LEMON SOUR CONQUERS
THAT HANGOVER HEADACHE

Annemarie Colbin, a holistic nutritionist and a wonderful mentor, swears by Mother Celestina's Tea for headaches associated with stress on the liver.

½ organic lemon
1¼ cup water
½ teaspoon honey or maple syrup (optional)

Wash the lemon rind. Juice the lemon, reserving the juice in a cup. Slice the juiced half in quarters and simmer in boiling water, covered, for 10 minutes. Strain the water into the cup with the juice. If too tart or too bitter, add the honey or maple syrup. Drink hot.

VISIONS OF SUGAR PLUMS

Japanese pickled plums, known as *umeboshi*, have remarkable medicinal qualities. Their powerful acidity has a paradoxical alkalinizing effect on the body, neutralizing fatigue and stimulating the digestion and promoting the elimination of toxins. This is the Far Eastern equivalent to both aspirin and apple; not only is it a potent hangover remedy for mornings after but an *umeboshi* a day is regarded as the best preventive medicine available.

Umeboshi plums are available in jars at Asian markets and natural-foods stores. They taste very salty. Japanese herbalists say the saltiness helps put the body back into balance by contracting the tissues that have overexpanded from too much alcohol. For a normal hangover, bite off about a quarter of a plum and keep it in your mouth until it dissolves. For a whopper hangover, herbalists recommend popping a whole plum in your mouth. Continue to suck on the pit for about an hour after the plum has dissolved.

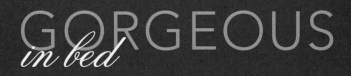

CHAPTER 04

GORGEOUS
in bed

IT'S IN THE BAG, BABY!

Caught with your pants down? Plotting a sleepover? Doing the walk of shame? Carry these essentials in your purse—*le* must for *le* morning after!

Breath mints—to freshen up your kisser

Clear nail polish—a fast fix for anything broken

Condoms—ladies' choice it is

Contact case and saline—to keep you bright-eyed

Crackberry—so you can email your date if you're late

Hairbrush, essential hair products, hair accessories— tame that mane

Hand lotion—blessed relief for chapped paws

Mirror compact—you're the fairest of them all

Nail file—lose the pointy Elvira edge

Sunglasses—they help you look more chic, less freak

Swarovski blinged-out Band Aids—go from blistered to bang-up

Tide to Go pens—butterfingers be gone

And in case of emergency keep a couple of tampons and some dental floss handy.

salacious sex: APHRODISIACS

We've all heard that certain foods rev up your sex drive. While some of these foods have been scientifically proven to stimulate our systems, the others seem a bit . . . funky. The following is a list of aphrodisiacs, some normal, and some, well, you be the judge. Figs, oysters, chocolate, asparagus, cheese, caviar, lobster, grapes, sardines, mushrooms, cinnamon, Spanish fly, and, last but not least, Rocky Mountain oysters (it doesn't matter what you call them—cooked right, testicles are a treat for some folks!) may increase your sexual prowess. You don't need to eat all these foods at once—lest you ruin a night of romance with some serious gas and indigestion!

THE GARDEN OF EATING

If you like to entice a man with more than just the fruits of your loins, have I got some sweet treats for you! Bear in mind that none of these foods are low in calories or sugar, but that's not exactly the point now is it? It's time for you to think outside the box (ahem) and introduce fun foods into your sex life:

- **Honey** will sweeten up your breasts and body and lead the bee right to your hive! Worried about stickiness? Trust me, it won't be on you long enough! For those who are carb-conscious, try **agave syrup**, which is derived from the nectar of the agave plant and looks and tastes like honey but is much lower in sugar.
- **Chocolate whipped cream** is the perfect topping for your sundae. Get the spray can, aim, and shoot!
- **Chocolate body paint:** Grab a paintbrush and run wild with your very own edible designs.
- If your man has Bill Clinton's charisma and charm, try sucking on a **candy cane** and head south of the Beltway for some executive hanky-panky.
- Try using **cake frosting** while playing naked Twister. Loser must lick!

Gorgeous Girl beware: If you battle yeast infections, keep these treats for external use only!

HERSHEY KISSES

There are delicious perks to eating chocolate. My favorite study compared heart rates and brain activity of people in their twenties who were given chocolate and then started macking. The kissing couples who ate chocolate got much more of a buzz and doubled their heart rates compared to couples who smooched without any chocolate. The moral of the story? Chocolate just may be better than kissing, but for maximum effect, try both!

ladies, start your engines:
SUPPLEMENTS

These natural solutions can boost a low sex drive, produce essential hormones, direct blood to your sex organs, soften your skin, and bolster your immune system to help discourage STDs.

- **B vitamins.** Your ability to react and respond to your leading man depends on how effectively your brain signals to your glands that it's time to initiate hormone production and the flow of blood to your sex organs. B vitamins are critical to the development of brain messengers for these signals.

- **Bioflavonoids.** Bioflavonoids keep blood vessels flexible and the uterus healthy. They also improve circulation to enhance whoopee potential. Bioflavonoids are found in a wide variety of plants, especially grapes.

- **Essential fatty acids.** EFAs are the building blocks of female sex hormone production. They also help your body store more of the fat-soluble vitamins (like E, D, and K) that keep you sexually active. In addition, they provide moisture and softness to the skin, eyes, vagina, and bladder. Borage, primrose, flaxseeds, fish oils, and wild Alaskan salmon are excellent sources of EFAs. (Read more about EFAs in Jiffy Lubing: Do You Need An Oil Change?, page 120.)

- **Vitamin E.** Found in olive oil, seeds and nuts, and organic butter, vitamin E can alleviate impotence and low sex drive. It protects your sex glands from free radicals that can damage proteins, DNA, and the lipids inside the cells.

IN ZINC

The human sense of smell, which depends on the mineral zinc, is an oft-overlooked element in primal passion. Pheromones—in this case, the individual biological scent your body produces—can drive your lover wild. They're detected subconsciously but are key in sexual excitement. Unfortunately, in today's smell-phobic society, the use of deodorants (and the contraceptive pill) seems to have interfered with our natural pheromone functions. So, to keep your lover attracted to the real you, try using natural deodorants with a tea tree oil base—they'll keep the bacteria at bay but let the true you shine through.

To tune in to your lover's pheromones, it's critical to make sure you're getting enough zinc-rich foods in your diet, including oysters and other shellfish, turkey, mushrooms, and seeds like sesame, sunflower, poppy, and pumpkin. Also, try sprouts, such as sunflower and alfalfa.

Zinc-rich foods also increase sexual function in women. Zinc supports healthy adrenal activity, which combats the negative effects of stress. Healthy adrenals translate to more energy, and because you'll feel less burned out by physical activity, you'll benefit from increased sexual stamina. Zinc bolsters your immune function, too, and may reduce your risk of contracting sexually transmitted diseases.

jiffy lubing:
DO YOU NEED AN OIL CHANGE?

So what to do about dry sex? Here are some simple remedies:

First and foremost, eating healthful fats is essential. If you've been eating poor-quality fats for years and you suddenly decide to clean out the riffraff, give your body *at least one year* to displace all the unhealthy fats with the healthy ones at the cellular level. Don't get discouraged. Remember that fat cells release toxins very slowly, so just give your body time. Even small changes in your diet will yield big results.

- Take at least 1–2 tablespoons of flaxseed oil every day.
- You can also alternate flaxseed oil with cod-liver oil to boost your immune system. Don't try just any old nasty-tasting fish oil, mind you; look for lemon-flavored oil, which doesn't have a hint of fishiness once it's refrigerated.
- For symptomatic relief, insert a wheat-germ-oil gelcap into the vagina; this remedy is safe and gentle enough to use even if you're prone to yeast infections. Wheat-germ oil is rich in vitamin E and will help re-create natural lubrication. You can insert it up to 1 hour before intercourse. As it warms up to your body temperature, the gelcap will dissolve and leave behind a silky residue. And it doesn't just feel good—it tastes good too! You can take wheat-germ oil orally as well.

PUTTING THE GAS MASK TO REST!

Let's face it, gals: Letting one rip in the middle of an intimate moment is embarrassing and a potential deal-breaker. Follow these steps to kick those unwanted stink-bombs out of the boudoir—for good.

- Take acidophilus capsules or powder every day, especially if you are on oral contraceptive pills and/or antibiotics. Make sure you take them with food. Acidophilus works to build "good bacteria" in your intestinal tract, which bulks up your bowel movements and enables them to pass through more quickly.
- Optimize your daily fiber intake. A high-fiber diet helps build "good bacteria" in your system, which in turn helps your body make digestive enzymes.
- Drink an adequate amount of water, herbal tea, or diluted juice to stay hydrated; at least 60 percent of constipation cases are due to dehydration. To figure out how much water you need, take your body weight in pounds and divide that number in half; that's how many ounces you'll need. For example, a 150-pound person would need 75 ounces of water, or about 9 glasses per day. For every caffeinated drink you have, add another glass of water to your daily needs. During exercise, drink 4 to 8 ounces of water every 20 minutes.
- Eating bitter, dark green leafy vegetables, as well as beets, will help stimulate the digestive process and facilitate elimination.

FRESH BOUQUET

Self-conscious about the way your vagina smells? Take some simple steps to improve the situation. First and foremost: Wear cotton undies, don't sit around in wet clothes, and skip the underwear at night. Let yourself air out and your vagina will repay you in kind. In the shower, use a very gentle cleanser and don't oversoap yourself, which can be very irritating to the delicate tissue in the area and can cause changes in pH balance that can worsen yeast infections.

When you're feeling not-so-fresh, you may be tempted to douche. I don't recommend it. All healthy vaginas contain some bacteria and other organisms called the vaginal flora. The normal acidity of the vagina keeps the amount of bacteria down. Douching can change this delicate balance by decreasing the acidity of the vagina—ultimately making a woman more prone to vaginal infections. Plus, douching can introduce new bacteria up into the uterus, fallopian tubes, and ovaries.

Last but not least, know your scent. If there's something amiss down there, and there haven't been any takers for your bouquet lately, hustle on over to your gyno's office and get things checked out. A change in odor that is reminiscent of last night's fish dinner could be caused by bacterial vaginosis (read on in this chapter for more information).

bacterial vaginosis:
THERE'S SOMETHING FISHY GOING ON

Bacterial vaginosis is an infection caused by an overgrowth of the bacteria that are normally present in the vagina. Although it is more common in women who are sexually active, it also occurs in women who are not sexually active (self-pleasuring doesn't count here!). Like yeast infections, the symptoms often include a discharge, which can have a fishy smell. Vaginosis can be treated with medication, either topical or oral, prescribed by your doctor. I also recommend that you take a heaping teaspoon of acidophilus powder to recalibrate your vaginal habitat and for long-term prevention.

PUNANI POWER

Kegel exercises are designed to help strengthen the pelvic floor. Keeping this muscle in tiptop shape will strengthen erections and improve orgasms. Giddyup!

Beginner: Baby Steps

1.   Clench your PC muscle and hold for 5 seconds; rest for 5 seconds. Repeat 10 times.
2.   Quickly clench your PC muscle and hold for 10 seconds; rest for 10 seconds and then repeat. Perform 3 sets and then take a 30-second break.
3.   Clench your PC muscle and hold for 30 seconds; rest for 30 seconds. Repeat 3 times.
4.   Repeat the first step and you're done for the day.

Intermediate: Glamma-Puss

1.   Clench your PC muscle and hold for 5 seconds; release. Repeat 10 times.
2.   Squeeze and release the muscle 10 times quickly. Do 3 sets.

3. Clench and release your PC muscle, alternating long counts of 10 with short counts of 10. Repeat 3 times.
4. Squeeze your PC muscle and hold it for as long as you can. Try to work your way up to 120 seconds. (Relax, that's only 2 minutes.)

Advanced: Ride 'Em, Cowgirl!

1. Fully squeeze and release your PC muscle over and over again. Begin with one set of 30; slowly work your way up to more than 100.
2. Squeeze your PC muscle as tightly as you possibly can. (Make sure it's only your PC muscle that you're clenching, not your PC and abdominals.) Hold it for 20 seconds, then rest for 30 seconds. Repeat 5 times.

antibiotics: INFECTIONS' FRIEND OR FOE?

We all know that antibiotics are a fast solution to nagging infections, but in the long run, they can cause more harm than good. I don't knock them altogether; there is a time and a place for antibiotics. But if you're using them once a year or more, your immune system needs a jump-start.

Often, the root cause of yeast infections is the overuse of antibiotics (either as an adult or as a child), birth control pills, a high-sugar diet, stress, or poor hygiene practices. The best way to treat the infections is through lifestyle change, because once you have a yeast infection you will always be prone to them. For vaginal yeast infections, stick to a whole-foods diet rich in fiber. Garlic, yogurt, and flaxseeds all help create a healthy gut environment, which makes it far more difficult for yeast to thrive.

If you are prone to sinus infections, invest in a Neti Pot. They resemble hobbit-sized teapots, which you fill with a saline solution and pour through your nasal cavities. Sounds unglamorous, but regular nasal lavage will treat sinus infection symptoms and provide much-needed relief without your having to resort to antibiotics and their resultant yeast infections. (See Troubleshooting: Yeast and Sinus Infections, page 196.)

THE PILL CAN BE A REAL PILL

The pill can deplete the body's stores of vitamin B_6, which is critical for healthy nerve function, water balance, and the production of serotonin and dopamine. Serotonin and dopamine are powerful neurotransmitters that help keep us happy and calm. Without them, we can become quite depressed, crave sugars, and may need antidepressants. If you are on the pill, take at least 50 mg of B_6 per day.

The pill can also exacerbate systemic yeast overgrowth. So, if you pop these hormones every day, supplement with probiotics, which promote healthy gut function and fight yeast overgrowth by sustaining the good bacteria in your system. This helps ensure that yeast levels do not get out of control. Everyone on the pill needs to take probiotics every day; powder or pills are fine, just aim for a count of eight billion per day.

A word to the wise: Use condoms regardless of whether you are taking the pill. There are tons of STDs out there, and slipping a raincoat on your man's johnson takes all of about five seconds (trust me, I've mastered it), so no excuses.

HERPES

Boosting the immune system with nutrients that have antiviral properties can help your body fight the good fight. Olive leaf extract, vitamin C, St. John's wort, and echinacea have a powerful effect on the body that help keep herpes symptoms at bay. L-lysine has also shown to be effective against herpes by improving the balance of nutrients necessary to reduce viral growth of the herpes virus.

Herpes Symptom Soothers

- **Olive leaf extract:** 500 mg (*Olea europaea* leaf standardized to 6 percent [30 mg] oleuropein); take 4 capsules every 3 hours, up to 16 a day.
- **L-lysine:** 500 mg; take 6 capsules twice per day.
- **Vitamin C:** 1,000 mg 3 times per day.
- **St. John's wort** (from *Hypericum perforatum* flowering herb 2.5 g): take 1 teaspoon diluted in a shot of water or juice.
- **Echinacea** (from *Echinacea purpurea* root 1:2 extract): 1 teaspoon diluted in a shot of water or juice.
- **Calcium lactate:** 250 mg twice per day.

Avoid soy, nuts and seeds, sugar, and alcohol during active herpes outbreaks. Sugar and alcohol will wear down your immune system, and soy, nuts, and seeds are very high in arginine, an amino acid that can counteract the effects of lysine. Lysine is an amino acid that suppresses the signs and symptoms of herpes.

DYSPLASIA AND GENITAL WARTS

For dysplasia and genital warts, use the protocol below from your first diagnosis until your next Pap smear, which should be done six months later. The protocol listed below should help normalize your cervical cells.

HPV Soothers

- **Beta carotene:** 50,000 IU per day for 6 months—make sure it's from a food-based formula.
- **Folic acid:** 20 mg per day for 6 months.
- **Echinacea:** 1 teaspoon of liquid extract (from *Echinacea purpurea* root 1:2 extract) diluted in a shot of water or juice; take once a day for 6 months.

Last but not least, don't forget to keep yourself updated on the most cutting-edge facts and figures about STDs by logging on to the American Social Health Association's Web site, www.ashastd.org. If you already have herpes or an STD, try visiting the online dating Web site www.mpwh.org. If you can't beat 'em, join 'em!

UTIs (URINARY TRACT INFECTIONS)

A UTI is an infection anywhere in the urinary tract. The urinary tract is the body's filtering system for the removal of liquid wastes. UTIs can be pesky and painful reminders that you've just indulged in a wild sexfest. Honeymooners out there, beware! To keep bacteria away from your urethra, make sure you pee after having sex and wipe yourself front to back. The same goes for bowel movements—clean yourself up well, because the bacteria that cause UTIs lives in your intestines, so pooping with poor hygiene can lead to a UTI. Fortunately, there are natural remedies that will treat your UTI and let you avoid using antibiotics.

Piss-Poor: Treatment for UTIs and Cystitis

D-Mannose powder: Take 1 teaspoon in water every three hours for the first two days. On day three, take 1 teaspoon three times per day. On day four, take just 1 teaspoon. The maintenance dose is 1 teaspoon per day. Drink a *lot* of water. D-mannose prevents *E. coli* bacteria from sticking to the bladder walls.

Cranberry concentrate (cranberry fruit juice concentrate in a 25:1 formulation): Take 2 tablets three or four times per day for acute infections and 1 tablet three or four times per day for chronic infections. Take 1 tablet three times per day as a maintenance dose.

Uva-ursi leaf (500 mg in a 4:1 extract): Take 2 tablets three or four times per day for acute infections and 1 tablet three or four times per day for chronic infections. Take 1 tablet three times per day as a maintenance dose.

PUT THE SWING IN HIS DING

Freshly ground flaxseeds are an especially good source of omega-3 fats for men. Flaxseeds are rich in lignans, the insoluble fibers that help protect against both breast and prostate cancers. Three tablespoons of flax meal provides 8 g of fiber, and it's easy to sprinkle on yogurt and ice cream and in protein smoothies, oatmeal, and salads. Fish and fish-oil supplements are also a wonderful source of omega-3s. If he eats wild cold-water fatty fish, like wild Alaskan salmon or sardines, three to five times per week, it will help promote circulation throughout his body—especially to all the crucial areas where every ounce of blood counts!

If you need to address your man's low sex drive, think zinc! Zinc helps make testosterone. About 25 mg per day is sufficient for a maintenance dose, but if your man eats a diet high in sugar and/or refined carbs, his zinc levels will probably be low (excess carbohydrates and starches naturally deplete the body's zinc reserves), so suggest 50 mg per day for about three months to get him up to speed.

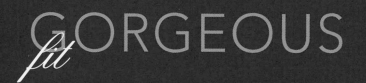

CHAPTER 05

fit GORGEOUS

FEELING FLABULOUS?

Finding something fun to do that will get your groove on and make you feel fabulous about your body is such a boost for your confidence. While the gym is a great place to get fit, consider more wicked ways to work it out:

Pole dancing: Great for the Gorgeous Girl who wants to add a little more sensuality into her life. Luckily it's a great workout too—it builds endurance, strength, and tones muscles, especially the core. No wonder strippers look so fit! Best yet, you can install a pole in your home to impress all your friends and neighbors.

Belly dancing: Belly dancing encompasses seductive dance moves with advanced fitness that can include floor gymnastics, back bends, poses, and stretches. Don some finger cymbals, shake your hips, and let your mind and body go with the flow.

Boot camp: Not for the timid or weak at heart. You'll need some serious determination and commitment for this very intense but completely worth it workout. Pounds will melt off as you lunge, run, do jumping jacks, pushups, and all kinds of imaginative and creative workouts that will get your energy soaring.

PLAYING HEART TO GET

There are many schools of thought on the best way to burn calories and fat. But the most efficient bang for your buck is, by far, cardio-vascular interval training coupled with strength training. While some of us thrive on long-distance endurance exercise, for most of us, that kind of exercise is simply too stressful on our bodies. In hunter-gatherer times, going to kill our dinner involved fast-action sprint-ing, and that is still the way our bodies work today. Long periods of a high-intensity workout elevate cortisol levels and help us break down muscle and store fat. If you've ever trained for an endurance event, you may notice you've packed on the pounds despite burning thousands of calories in training. Well now you can eliminate that from happening, and for good. If you're an adrenaline junkie, not to worry. These exercises will kick your arse so hard you won't feel like you're missing anything! And if you hate to work out in the first place, then relish in the fact that there's a touch of downtime built into the following routines.

interval training: PEAKS AND VALLEYS

Start by strapping on a heart-rate monitor. After a 10-minute warm-up, exercise at a higher intensity but at a pace you could maintain for the entire workout. Then, push yourself hard for one minute, with a short burst of activity you couldn't do for longer than a minute. Recover for three minutes, getting your heart rate back down to baseline, and then increase the intensity again. Complete eight cycles of three minutes aerobic/recovery and one minute anaerobic exercise. Then cool down for a minimum of five minutes and stretch afterward. If you are a beginner, you can shorten the interval times, or the amount of intervals completed, and gradually build up. Do this two to three times per week to see gains in your fitness levels.

BABY STEPS

For all of you who love walking for exercise, then bully for you! Walking produces far less injuries than other forms of exercise, requires little to no fitness equipment (save for a pair of sassy sneaks), is free of charge, and gives you changing scenery throughout your workout. Talk about an antidote for boredom! Now here's the kicker: For best results you've got to walk without interruption and throw in some hills for resistance training. So march yourself up and down the stairs for some tush-trimming fitness, walk up hills to tone your calves and slim your thighs, and mix it all up to strengthen your heart. Carrying groceries, parking the car far away from the store, taking the stairs—all of these are giant steps in reaching your fitness goals.

A great motivational tool is a pedometer, and luckily iPods and cell phones have them built right in! For best results aim for a count of six to ten thousand steps per day, the equivalent of walking three to five miles.

THE RIGHT TO BARE ARMS

To keep your arms strapless-gown ready, de-flabbed, firmed, and toned, you'll need to add strength training two to three times per week to your cardio routine. Adding definition to your arms will not only help your body burn fat better and keep you jiggle-free, but you'll also look great when swimsuit season comes along. The best news is that upper-body muscles usually respond quickly to resistance training because they don't get the same wear and tear as our legs typically do. Bear this in mind, however: When getting your arms lean and mean, you may need to slim down a bit if you happen to store body fat in your arms; otherwise, the muscle you are building will be hidden under layers of fat. Whatever strength exercises you choose, be sure to fatigue your muscles after ten to twelve repetitions, and do three sets of repetitions total. Initially, you may only be able to do a few repetitions, but over time you'll build up your strength. Pushups, bicep curls, tricep dips and kickbacks, and bench presses will all do the trick!

AB FAB

To get those strong, flat, fierce abdominal muscles, a girl can't live by crunches alone. Strong abs don't actually start in your gym; they start in your kitchen. So, to get the best results, you'll need to commit to a steadfast plan of good nutrition, aerobic exercise, and core-specific strengthening. The dedication is demanding but the payoff is big. Rope in a friend, if you can, so you have a built-in support system to reaching your goals.

Choose three exercises from the following list, and do four to five sets of ten to twelve repetitions each, two to three times per week:

- Bicycle crunches
- Crunches on a physio ball
- Plank pose (hold for three sets of one-minute poses)
- Swiss ball reverse crunches
- Medicine ball throws on Swiss ball

OUT-BURSTS

Mixing up your workouts by alternating bursts of energy with periods of rest not only turns your workout into a "playout," but also gives your body the most efficient workout possible. Sprinting actually raises your level of human growth hormone, so you build muscle and burn more fat. So, for you busy bees out there who barely have time to squeeze in slimnastics, try some timesaving activities to get your body moving fast and furious.

Jumping rope, squats, lunges, riding a stationary bike, running, or rollerblading are all excellent ways to rock your body. Interval training can be done with any type of exercise, so don't forget to mix and match your workouts, otherwise your body will quickly adjust to its workload. Keep challenging yourself every four weeks with new routines. And wear a heart rate monitor so that you know you're reaching your goals.

BURN, BABY, BURN

Try to think of exercise as an opportunity instead of a punishment. It is a privilege to be physically able to do what we want, when we want. So the trick is to do things you really enjoy that will also give you results. Be mindful of the difference between activity and exercise: Activity encompasses the day-to-day movements that are part of your routine. Gardening, carrying groceries, getting the paper, climbing the stairs in your home—doing those every day may initially give your metabolism and derriere a boost, but after a few months of repetition you'll need to add new challenges to the mix. Get a workout partner or invest in a personal trainer to keep you motivated and help you reach your fitness goals. And make sure you reward yourself for reaching your goals.

NO GYM? NO SWEAT!

You don't need a gym to get fit. There's simply no excuse for not getting your rear in gear. Grab a friend or personal trainer, and get going!

Indoor Workouts

- Exercise bands
- Physio ball
- Hand weights
- Lunges and squats
- Run up and down the stairs in your building; if you are traveling take the hotel stairs while carrying your briefcase
- Walk or run on a treadmill or ride a stationery bike
- Roller skating
- Ice skating
- Yoga or Pilates

Outdoor Workouts

- Walk, run, or go for a bike ride
- Strap on some rollerblades
- Triceps dips on a park bench
- Lunges and squats
- Pull-ups at the playground
- Push-ups
- Swimming

GET YOUR RUMP READY FOR A HUMP

Wondering if there are any fast fixes to help you go from dumpy to date-worthy? A burst of intense exercise coupled with some clean eating will give you the boost you need to feel great on a date. Incorporate these exercises a minimum of two weeks prior to your big day:

Single-leg squats—three sets of 15 repetitions
Reverse lunges—three sets of 15 repetitions
Squats—three sets of 15 repetitions
Shoulder bridge butt squeezes—three sets of 10 repetitions
Triceps dips—three sets of 10 repetitions
Push-ups—three sets of 10 repetitions
Plank position—hold for three sets of 1-minute poses

Make sure you add dumbbells to your routine once you get over the initial hump (pun intended) so that your strength and fitness levels keep improving. Also make sure you do at least three 30-minute sessions of interval training per week to burn some serious calories and fat.

Visualize a stronger and leaner version of yourself as you work out and you'll reach your goal in no time.

CHAPTER 06

GORGEOUS
blues

FAKE IT TILL YOU MAKE IT

There's a saying that goes: Some days you're the bug, and some days you're the windshield. When you feel like the bug, what's the best way to get through the tough times? Fake it till you make it. Develop a mantra for yourself and repeat it whenever you feel anxious. It can be as simple as "Everything's going to be okay" or "I am stronger than I think." Our cells register both negative and positive messages at the cellular level, so much so that our thoughts can influence the way our DNA expresses illness during times of depression, or how it leaves those genes dormant during times of happiness. Take charge of your health first by starting with the language you use to express your thoughts. Over time, repeating encouraging words will help change your way of thinking about yourself, and your body will pay you in kind by hooking on to the silver lining you are projecting into the universe. Not only that, but your mind will also start to believe all the loving, kind, and gentle words you are feeding it. So embrace yourself, hold your chin up high, and remind yourself who's in charge here—you're gonna make it after all.

THAT'S THE SPIRIT!

Whether your daily rituals include a heavenly cup of something hot, a run in the park, a yoga session, or a conversation with your best friend, carve out time in your day for you. Downtime that quiets the mind and feeds the soul is essential for juicing up our internal batteries, and it gives us pleasure and perspective in life.

Your body registers happiness and trauma at the cellular level; clearing out internal clutter and balancing your energy is essential for sustaining balance and inner harmony.

FOR EVERY SEASON . . .

Ever notice that you have seasons for certain illnesses? Some Gorgeous Gals routinely suffer from winter respiratory infections while others are slaves to the summer cold. Springtime is notorious for allergies, while fall brings on seasonal affective disorder, depression, and sore throats. Whatever your affliction, the remedy is often in the kitchen. Read on for a few stellar ideas that will keep your immune system humming. . . .

Spring Cleaning

To treat seasonal allergies, give your adrenal glands some lovin'. Nettles help prevent the body from making inflammatory chemicals known as prostaglandins. Quercetin is used for its antihistamine and anti-inflammatory properties. Also make sure you eat plenty of protein and get adequate rest and hydration.

Borage oil	240 mg twice daily, with food
Quercitin	1,200 mg three times daily, with food
Nettles	1,200 mg three times daily, with food
MSM	1,000 mg three times daily, with food
Licorice	(from *Glycyrrhiza glabra* root 2.5 g) 1 teaspoon of liquid tincture diluted in 1 ounce of water

FOR EVERY SEASON . . .

Summer Lovin'

Afraid of the sun, you say? Think that you're going to get cancer every time a ray of sun hits your face? Then think again, my fair young lassies! Believe it or not, more cancers are caused from low vitamin D levels then from direct sun exposure itself. So get yourself some luminescence at least three times per week for a minimum of fifteen minutes each time—up to thirty minutes if you have a very dark complexion. That's right ladies—direct sunlight, sans sunscreen, on your Gorgeous bod. This will boost your immune function and help fight those summer colds. It's also important to take some extra vitamin C, as the sun depletes our body's supply within about twenty minutes of exposure. In terms of diet, make sure you eat antioxidant-rich foods, which can act as an internal sunscreen, including wild Alaskan salmon.

Sun-Goddess Supplements

Vitamin C	500 mg twice per day, with food
Green tea extract	300 mg per day, with food
Astaxanthin	4 mg per day, with food

FOR EVERY SEASON . . .

Fall in Love . . . with Vitamin D

To help you skip through the fall without any depression or seasonal affective disorder, get your blood tested for vitamin D levels. The new requirements state that optimal levels for vitamin D should be 60 ng/dL. If you can't be bothered to get to the doctor's office or are skittish when it comes to needles, take at least 2,000 IU per day of vitamin D to keep your levels up throughout the winter. Also, make sure you take omega-3 fatty acids to boost your serotonin levels; 2,000–4,000 mg per day should do the trick.

FOR EVERY SEASON . . .

Winter Colds: An Ounce of Prevention . . .

To cruise through the winter cold-free, keep up with a healthy daily diet and supplement regime. Be judicious about the sugar you consume, lest you wipe out your immune system completely. Instead, make sure you get plenty of vitamin A–rich foods, which support lung health, like sweet potatoes, winter squash, and carrots, as well as dark green leafy vegetables. Also, try taking a daily shot of wheatgrass or a powdered green-vegetable drink mixed with water. You may cringe at the thought at first, but after a month or so you'll feel so fabulous you'll wonder how you ever lived without it! Other heavenly immunization tools for your arsenal:

Andrographis	400 mg per day (Andrographis herb 10:1 extract from *Andrographis paniculata* herb 1.0 g)
Maitake D	2 capsules twice per day (each capsule should contain 150 mg maitake mushroom powder and 10 mg maitake standardized extract)
Echinacea	1 teaspoon per day (from *Echinacea purpurea* root 2.5 g)
Calcium lactate	250 mg twice per day

For chronic lung conditions and respiratory problems, take a dropperful of micellized vitamin A once per week. Mix it with a shot of pomegranate or grape juice, as it tastes pretty bitter!

FIND YOUR RHYTHM

Feel like you've missed a beat? Going through PMS and then not getting your period can drive any Gorgeous Girl to the brink. Many women want some level of predictability in their lives and reach for the pill when irregularity strikes. However, the pill will never get to the root of the problem. So to keep your rhythm, try the following:

- Eat as cleanly as possible, and make sure you get plenty of beneficial fats in your diet: raw nuts and seeds, fresh avocado, olive oil, and ground flaxseeds. Without the right types of fats or enough fats, our bodies can't manufacture our hormones properly. Steer clear of hydrogenated oils, margarine, and fried foods.
- Add these hormone-balancing supplements to your regime (you'll need to stick with these for six months to see a difference):

Chaste tree*	(Chaste tree fruit 6:1 extract from *Vitex agnus-castus* fruit 500 mg) 240 mg, first thing in the morning
Evening primrose oil	1,000 mg twice per day, with food

Gorgeous Girl beware! DO NOT take chaste tree if you are on the pill, as it will counteract its efficacy.

PMS

If you think PMS stands for Putting up with Men's Shit, you definitely need some nutritional support! The major causes of PMS are hormonal imbalances, low blood sugar, poor liver detoxification, and an imbalance of nutrients.

The first step in bidding adieu to PMS is to eat your protein. Protein supports the liver, which detoxifies estrogen as it fluctuates through your system. Plus, it balances your hormones and stabilizes your blood sugar. At least two out of three meals per day should contain three or more ounces of protein, such as lean meats, poultry, eggs, or fish. Next, eliminate or minimize caffeinated and chemical-laden beverages such as diet sodas, coffee, and black tea, and flush your body with filtered water and antioxidant-rich green or white teas. Be sure to avoid artificial sweeteners. These can wreak just as much havoc on your blood sugar as regular table sugar. The sweet taste tricks your brain into believing that it has eaten something sweet, prompting the same rise in blood sugar as from regular sugar, which can promote weight gain. And it gets worse: Artificial sweeteners also interfere with the uptake of serotonin and dopamine in the brain—two neurotransmitters that give us a happy, contented feeling. Ultimately, artificial sweeteners can cause, or worsen, depression.

PUMPING IRON

If you're feeling more down than usual, notice spoon-shaped fingernails and toenails, or have heavy bleeding with menstrual cycles, head over to your doctor's office to test for anemia. Sensitivity to cold, PMS, menstrual clots, mental sluggishness, and depression have all been linked to anemia. Antacids and drugs are often culprits, and exercise-induced anemia is becoming more and more common.

What's the fastest way to increase your iron stores? Eating organic beef and liver, which have the highest iron content in the most bioavailable form for your body. Incorporate red kidney beans, spinach, collard and mustard greens, and dark green salad into your diet as well. If you're vegetarian or just don't enjoy eating beef and liver, take both iron and vitamin B_{12} supplements with folic acid (anemics often lack vitamin B_{12}).

Make sure to eat your meat with a vitamin C source (tomatoes, tomato sauce, peppers, baked potatoes with the skin) or take a vitamin C supplement with your iron to facilitate absorption. Lastly, have a shot of wheatgrass every day. Studies have shown that taking chlorophyll (think dark green leafy vegetables) with iron increases red blood cells and blood hemoglobin faster than just taking iron alone.

CHAPTER 07

GORGEOUS
troubleshooting

ACNE, BUTTNE, AND BACKNE

Supplements

Zinc	50 mg per day for three to four months; then decrease dosage to 25 mg per day for maintenance
Probiotics	8–16 billion per day, in either powdered or capsule form
Vitamin A	25,000 IU for one month; then 5,000 IU per day as a maintenance dose; capsules made from fish oil are quite effective.
Omega-3s	1,000 mg twice per day
Borage oil (GLA)	240 mg twice per day
Vitamin C	500 mg twice per day
Tea tree oil	Apply topically once or twice per day to spot-treat blemishes.

Nutritional Approaches

This protocol works beautifully for all skin types, because the omega-3s and the GLA will regulate your oil production. For best results, eliminate sugar, wine, and beer, which will all contribute to breakouts and deplete your body's zinc stores. Also, keep a tight rein on the bread and yeasty foods you eat, which can also worsen the problem. Try to practice yoga once per week for stress management as well.

ALL BACKED UP?

Supplements

Magnesium	400 mg twice per day on an empty stomach
Probiotics	8–16 billion per day
Pancreatic enzymes	160 mg Pancreatin 5X (each capsule should contain 20,000 USP units of amylase and protease and 1,600 USP units of lipase) per meal
Betaine hydrochloride	200 mg per meal
Spanish black radish	1 tablet three times per day

Nutritional Approaches

Feeling constipated can be a frustrating experience. The good news is that some basic nutritional changes in your diet will usually do the trick and get you right as rain. Check in with yourself and make sure you are hydrated. Your basic water needs are half your body weight in ounces per day—more if you work out and/or drink caffeinated beverages. Be sure to increase your fiber intake by adding 2 to 3 tablespoons of freshly ground flaxseeds into your oatmeal, yogurt, cottage cheese, or juice. The fiber content in the flaxseeds will help your body make digestive enzymes and will also regulate your bowel movements. And keep your intake of flour products on the low side since flour plus water makes paste.

ALLERGIES (SEASONAL OR DIETARY)

Supplements for Seasonal Allergies

Borage oil (GLA)	250 mg twice per day
Omega-3s	1,000 mg twice per day
Quercetin	500 mg twice per day
Astragalus root	200 mg twice per day
Echinacea root	100 mg twice per day

Supplements for Dietary Allergies

Take the protocol listed above and add:

L-glutamine	5,000 mg per day in powdered form, diluted into water
Probiotics	8–16 billion per day

Nutritional Approaches

Eliminate wheat, cheese, and milk, which are three of the most common allergens in our diet today and which can exacerbate both food and seasonal allergies. Plain yogurt has numerous health benefits, so go for it! Try buckwheat (soba) noodles or rice-based cellophane noodles instead of flour-based pasta. Drink plenty of nettle tea, which can also decrease the allergenic response. Quercetin is known for its ability to block the release of histamines, thereby preventing allergy symptoms like swollen nasal passages, congestion, sneezing, watery eyes, and itchiness in the eyes and nose.

BONE HEALTH

Supplements

Vitamin D	2,000 IU per day
Calcium	1,000 mg per day on an empty stomach
Magnesium	400 mg per day on an empty stomach
Omega-3s	1,000 mg per day

Also take a multivitamin or trace mineral supplement that contains 25 mg zinc, 2 mg copper, 5 mg boron, and 150 mcg of vitamin K.

Nutritional Approaches

If there's a history of osteoporosis in your family, get a head start on your bone health right now. Weight training two or three times per week is important for building bones. Also, get your vitamin D status checked yearly; your blood test should show a level of 60 ng/dL or greater. A diet rich in whole foods that includes adequate protein, sesame seeds or tahini, almonds, and dark green leafy vegetables is imperative. Whether or not you consume dairy, take vitamin D supplements. Try to get fifteen minutes of sunshine at least three days per week. You must expose as much of your skin as possible without any sunscreen to reap the benefits—wearing as little as SPF-8 sunscreen decreases the body's ability to make vitamin D by 95 percent!

BRITTLE NAILS

Supplements

MSM	1,000 mg three times per day
Calcium	1,000 mg per day
Magnesium	400–800 mg per day
Horsetail	1 teaspoon of liquid extract per day (from *Equisetum arvense* herb 2.5 g) diluted in water

Nutritional Approaches

Nails are composed of protein, so make sure you eat enough protein each day, as well as essential fatty acids and calcium-rich foods. To pamper your nails, try rubbing olive or coconut oil into the cuticle and nail bed each night. If you have vertical ridges or dark lines down the nails, get your thyroid checked. If you have toenail fungus, try putting tea tree oil directly on top of the nails and under the nail bed. Last but not least, every now and then, take a break from using nail polish. Long-term nail polish use can cause dry, brittle nails. Go for the sexy look of naked nails while allowing them to come up for air.

CARPAL TUNNEL SYNDROME

Carpal tunnel syndrome (CTS) can be a real drag. Taking the pill and pregnancy both increase the risk of CTS, and so does excess time spent using your computer keyboard, and yes—even emailing on your Crackberry! The numbness occurs when the median nerve between your thumb and first two fingers is compressed during repetitive motions of your hand and wrist. Signals get short-circuited along the nerves, making it feel like your hands have fallen asleep. Splinting, heat, and cold can help relieve your symptoms. And you should also pop some extra supplements.

Supplements

B$_6$	50–100 mg per day
B complex	50 mg per day
St. John's wort	1 teaspoon per day (1:2 extract from *Hypericum perforatum* flowering herb 2.5 g)
Bromelain	1,000 mg three times per day
Circumin	500 mg per day

Nutritional Approaches

Stay on this protocol for a minimum of twelve weeks, or until you are fully healed. Make your workstation more ergonomically correct and avoid yoga poses or spin classes that put extra stress on your wrist.

COLDS AND FLUS

You know when you've got a cold coming on. Your eyes get a little glassy, there's a tickle in the back of your throat, your head aches, and you want to crawl right back into bed. The good news is that if you're lucky enough to catch it in time and nip it in the bud, you can prevent a cold from coming on, or at least shorten its duration.

Supplements

Vitamin C	Acute: 250 mg every hour. Maintenance: 500 mg twice per day
Echinacea	Acute: 1 teaspoon (from *Echinacea purpurea* root 2.5 g) three times per day. Maintenance: 1 teaspoon once or twice per day
Olive leaf extract	Two 500 mg capsules three times per day
Maitake D	Two capsules twice per day (1 capsule should contain 150 mg maitake mushroom powder and 10 mg maitake standardized extract)
Micellized vitamin A	For upper-respiratory-tract infections, take 1 dropperful per day, mixed into a shot of juice, for one week. For long-term prevention, take 1 dropperful once per week

MORE COLD AND FLU REMEDIES

Echinacea purpurea helps boost your white blood cell count and has natural antiviral properties. The liquid variety is much more effective because it is absorbed much more easily than the tablet form. Gargle with it when you have a sore throat to kill bacteria in the mouth and throat. Buy a brand with a minimum of 1.0 mg/ml of alkylamides for optimal strength and quality. Alkylamides enhance immune-system function, boost white blood cell count, support respiratory function, and help cleanse the lymphatic system. Good, potent echinacea should temporarily make your tongue feel numb and your mouth salivate; this tells you that active compounds are present.

Drink 8 to 16 ounces of clear liquids every hour. Herbal teas, chicken broth, miso soup, or diluted juices help flush out the bacteria and mucus from your body. Try eating a whole clove of garlic chopped up and mixed with 1 teaspoon of raw honey. Suck on zinc lozenges. Eat plenty of orange and dark green vegetables, which are rich in vitamin A.

If your system is really stubborn and these supplements aren't working fast enough, kick it up a notch with some freshly juiced veggies (especially chlorophyll-rich green ones)—they clear out the lymphatic system and have antibacterial benefits.

CONSTIPATION, GAS, AND BLOATING

Supplements

Magnesium	400 mg twice per day on an empty stomach
Probiotics	8–16 billion per day
Pancreatic enzymes	Take per meal: 160 mg Pancreatin 5X with 20,000 USP units of amylase and protease and 1,600 USP units of lipase
Betaine hydrochloride	200 mg per meal
Spanish black radish	1 tablet three times per day

Nutritional Approaches

Try these food-combining principles, which can really lighten the workload of the digestive tract: Eat all fruit first thing in the morning, on an empty stomach, half an hour before your breakfast. At meals, combine protein with vegetables and fat or carbohydrates with vegetables and fat, but do not combine protein with carbohydrates. Examples of a meal could be a salad, steak, and sautéed spinach, or beans, brown rice, and veggies. Also make sure to incorporate 2 to 3 tablespoons of freshly ground flaxseeds into your oatmeal, yogurt, cottage cheese, or juice. The fiber content in the flaxseeds will help your body make digestive enzymes and will also regulate your bowel movements.

GUTS AND GLORY

Many of us ladies have gluten sensitivities. If the word itself sends you running to the bathroom, you've got it bad and that ain't good. But try to think of your predisposition as an opportunity. Luckily, all the carb-counters out there have paved the way for going gluten-free. And it's another great reason to eat more plant-based foods and less food manufactured in plants. Do yourself a favor and check out a superbly hip guide to living well through gluten-free eating: www.glutenfreegirl.blogspot.com. Heartfelt writing and delicious recipes will whet your whistle and convert even the greatest skeptics. A little self-love and safe eating can do wonders for the soul and the belly.

And to heal yourself from within, don't forget to pop your probiotics, L-glutamine, and omega-3s.

DANDRUFF

Supplements

Probiotics	1 capsule (8 billion) twice per day for 1 month; 1 capsule per day for maintenance
Garlic	1 capsule per day (should contain 1 bulb per capsule)
Borage oil	2 capsules twice per day for 1 month; then 1 capsule twice per day for maintenance (1 capsule should contain 240 mg)
Spanish black radish	1 capsule three times per day

Nutritional Approaches

Dandruff is often an indication that your system contains a high amount of yeast, so limit your intake of sugar, yeasted foods, and foods that have trace amounts of fungus or mold: pasta, bread, cheese, sweets, mushrooms, soy sauce, vinegar, wine, and peanuts.

DEPRESSION

Supplements

Omega-3s	9,000–12,000 mg per day, with meals, in either liquid or capsule form
Inositol	Start with 1 teaspoon mixed in water three times per day. For severe depression, take 2 teaspoons three times daily.
Folic acid	2 mg per day
St. John's wort	1 teaspoon of liquid tincture (from *Hypericum perforatum* flowering herb 2.5 g) at bedtime

Nutritional Approaches

Depression is often associated with insulin resistance, so don't eat too many sugars, even if you crave them. Try to get a balance of protein, healthy fats, and complex carbohydrates at each meal to offset cravings and stabilize your blood sugar. Make sure you get your rear in gear and head to the gym for at least thirty minutes per day. Exercise is nature's antidepressant; it naturally raises your serotonin levels. Also make sure you get some fresh air and sunlight on a daily basis.

Gorgeous Girl beware! DO NOT take St. John's wort with 5-HTP, as it can cause serotonin syndrome, a potentially lethal syndrome.

DIARRHEA

Supplements

L-glutamine powder	1 teaspoon mixed into water every 3 hours
Probiotics	1 capsule or 1 teaspoon powder (8 billion) every 3 hours
Omega-3s	1,000–2,000 mg per day
Boswellia extract	300 mg two to four times per day
Oil of oregano	For food poisoning, take 1 drop in 8 ounces of water or tomato juice three times per day until symptoms resolve

Nutritional Approaches

Try the BRATT diet: bananas, white rice, applesauce, tea, and toast. These will all help bind you up and slow the pace of your intestinal spasms. Clear broths, and steamed chicken and fish, should work as well. Drink plenty of fluids to rehydrate yourself; chamomile and peppermint tea are both gentle and soothing. Also beef up your fiber intake with 2 to 3 tablespoons of ground flaxseeds each day. For colitis, IBS, Crohn's disease, or a more serious condition, visit www.scdiet.org and www.scdiet.com for incredible nutritional support with a gluten-free diet.

DRY SKIN

Supplements

Evening primrose oil	3,000 mg per day
Omega-3s	6,000 mg per day

Nutritional Approaches

Add flaxseed oil liberally to meals to act as an internal moisturizer. Make sure you bathe in warm, not hot, water so you don't overdry your skin. Keep coconut or olive oil in a spray bottle and apply it to damp skin after a shower. These oils are rich in natural emollients and will lock in moisture. A good rule of thumb: If you won't eat it, don't put it on your skin! Also make sure to get your thyroid checked out; dry skin can be a sign of an underactive thyroid. Use a humidifier (or even a pan of water placed near a radiator) to humidify your environment, especially in winter. This helps to reduce the amount of moisture lost from the skin through evaporation.

ENVIRONMENTAL TOXICITIES

Supplements

Lipoic acid	300 mg per day, with food
L-cysteine	1,000 mg per day
Glutathione	1,000 mg per day
Taurine	1,000 mg per day
MSM	1,000 mg per day

Nutritional Approaches

With the abundance of chemicals we are exposed to on a daily basis, it's important to protect your body with a nutritional suit of armor. The better nourished you are, the better your chances of fighting the good fight against toxins. Eating plenty of dark green leafy vegetables and drinking vegetable juices naturally facilitates your body's ability to remove toxins. Eating 8 to 12 ounces per day of protein is also an essential component of daily detoxification. If you are considering fasting, make sure you build yourself up for a few months beforehand with clean eating and supplements, otherwise, you could end up feeling worse and leave your body quite depleted.

FIBROCYSTIC BREASTS

Supplements

DIM	200 mg per day
Chaste tree*	4 tablets per day (from *Vitex agnus-castus* fruit 500 mg)
Evening primrose oil	2,000 mg per day
Milk thistle	150 mg twice per day
Spanish black radish	1 tablet with meals

Nutritional Approaches

The best thing you can do for painful breasts is to clear caffeine from your diet. Caffeine can greatly influence premenstrual breast tenderness. Drink plenty of water and limit high-salt foods so your breasts won't feel like two watermelons attached to your torso. Add 2 to 3 tablespoons of ground flaxseeds to your daily diet by tossing them into your oatmeal, yogurt, cottage cheese, salads, or a protein smoothie. After your period is finished each month, give yourself a breast self-examination, so you know your own lumpiness. Better yet, have your partner do it, which can be much more fun!

Gorgeous Girl beware! DO NOT take chaste tree if you are on the pill.

HANGOVERS

Supplements the Night Before

Milk thistle	300 mg
Schisandra	1 teaspoon of liquid tincture (250 mg)
DMAE	200 mg
Vitamin B$_6$	50 mg

Supplements the Morning After

Magnesium	400 mg as a rescue remedy
N-acetyl cysteine	1,000 mg
MSM	Start with 1,500 mg; after an hour, add another 1,500 mg if you feel you need extra support
L-glutamine	5,000 mg of powder dissolved in water for a sour stomach

Nutritional Approaches

Make sure you eat while you drink; drinking on an empty stomach is a fast ride on the expressway to a hangover. (Please refer back to Chapter 3, "Drinking Gorgeous," for a more in-depth discussion.) Fight alcohol-induced dehydration by alternating boozy cocktails with water or club soda with lemon. Drink tomato juice and eat crackers with raw honey the morning after to help your body metabolize the alcohol in your system.

HERPES

Supplements

Olive leaf extract	2,000 mg every 3 hours
L-lysine	3,000 mg capsules twice per day
Vitamin C	1,000 mg three times per day
Calcium lactate	250 mg twice per day
St. John's wort*	(from *Hypericum perforatum* flowering herb 2.5 gm) 1 teaspoon once per day diluted in a shot of water or juice
Echinacea	(from *Echinacea purpurea* root 1:2 extract) 1 teaspoon per day diluted in a shot of water or juice

Nutritional Approaches

Steer clear of nuts and nut butters, as well as all soy products. These foods are very high in arginine, which can exacerbate a herpes outbreak. Also avoid excess alcohol and sugar, which can suppress the immune system.

*Gorgeous Girl beware! re: St. John's Wort from page 169.

HIGH CHOLESTEROL

Supplements

Red yeast rice	1,200 mg twice per day
Omega-3s	3,000 mg twice per day
A-F betafood	3 tablets twice per day
B complex	50 mg per day

Nutritional Approaches

Diet-wise, limit or avoid the consumption of flour-based products, processed foods, and baked goods. In other words, anything white: white flour, white rice, muffins, pancakes, scones, donuts, sugar cereals, bagels, cookies, cakes . . . you get my drift. These foods are the culprits of heart disease, which is frequently termed "white-flour disease." These foods will raise your triglycerides as well, increasing your risk of heart disease. Incorporate wild Alaskan salmon, anchovies, sardines, fresh fruits and veggies, steel-cut oats, legumes, nuts, seeds, eggs (yes, even the yolks), olive oil, and a daily shot of pomegranate juice.

HIGH CORTISOL LEVELS

Supplements

Omega-3s	1,000 mg twice per day
Phosphatidylserine	300 mg at bedtime
Licorice root	(from *Glycyrrhiza glabra* root 2.5 g)
	First thing in the morning, take
	1 teaspoon of liquid tincture diluted in
	1 ounce of water
Ashwagandha root	(from *Withania somnifera* root 2.5 g)
	First thing in the morning, take
	1 teaspoon of liquid tincture diluted
	in 1 ounce of water

Nutritional Approaches

Have your doctor check your DHEA (dehydroepiandrosterone) levels. DHEA is a hormone that is made by the adrenal glands and is easily converted into other hormones, especially estrogen and testosterone. Low DHEA can cause hormonal and sleep disturbances, and high cortisol often lowers DHEA. Now is the time to try some deep breathing and relaxation techniques, which will also lower your cortisol levels. The same goes for yoga; even 10 minutes a day will help lower your cortisol levels.

INSOMNIA AND POOR SLEEP

Supplements

L-theanine	200 mg one hour before bedtime
GABA	550 mg one hour before bedtime
5-HTP	300 mg per day

Nutritional Approaches

Avoid sugar and alcohol before bed, as they cause fluctuations in your blood sugar levels and, ultimately, disrupt your sleep. Also check in with yourself about that caffeine habit of yours; even one cup of coffee in the morning can affect your sleep cycle that evening. A couple of hours before bed, eat a snack consisting of protein and some fruit; this combination will help your body make serotonin and melatonin, which should keep you slumbering all night. Sleep tight!

LIVER DETOX

Supplements

Lipoic acid	300–600 mg per day
Phosphatidyl choline	1200 mg per day, with food
Aqueous selenium	200 mcg per day
Milk thistle	300 mg per day

Nutritional Approaches

If your liver is on the lethargic side, you may be suffering from PMS, constipation, poor digestion of foods, dark brown circles under the eyes, allergies, and headaches. To give yourself the solid gold daily cure, eat plenty of dark green leafy vegetables, beets, carrots, artichokes, fennel, Brussels sprouts, dandelion greens, dandelion tea, and high-quality proteins. Think of this as feng shui for your liver, as it will remove all the internal cellular debris lurking in there!

LOW ENERGY

Supplements

Licorice root	(from *Glycyrrhiza glabra* root 2.5 g) First thing in the morning, take 1 teaspoon of liquid tincture diluted in 1 ounce of water
Ashwagandha root	(from *Withania somnifera* root 2.5 g) First thing in the morning, take 1 teaspoon of liquid tincture diluted in 1 ounce of water
L-carnitine	1,000 mg three times per day
Magnesium	400 mg twice per day
Lipoic acid	300 mg per day
CoQ10	100 mg twice per day

Nutritional Approaches

First and foremost, get your thyroid and mercury levels checked to rule out any organic causes. Check in with yourself and see what environmental stressors could be causing you to feel wiped out. Scoot on over to your fave yoga studio and get busy with some sun salutations and downward dogs. You'll be amazed at your energy level afterward! Also keep your caffeine intake to a minimum; it will only give you a temporary energy fix.

MENSTRUAL CRAMPS

Supplements

Cramp bark	(from *Viburnum opulus* bark 2.5 g) 1 teaspoon liquid tincture diluted in juice. Begin taking it the week before your period, and continue during your period as needed.
Magnesium	400 mg twice per day
Calcium lactate	250 mg every 3 hours while cramps are active
Evening primrose oil	3,000 mg per day

Nutritional Approaches

Eat 3 to 4 ounces of protein at each meal, especially the week before your period. Protein supports liver function and will help your body metabolize your hormones. Steer clear of any and all hydrogenated oils, which can generate severe inflammation that will aggravate menstrual cramps. Also avoid too much booze, which can temporarily alleviate cramps but will worsen them when the alcohol has worn off. If you need to take anti-inflammatory drugs for the pain, also take 1 heaping teaspoon of L-glutamine powder with water to avoid irritating the lining of your stomach.

MERCURY TOXICITY

Supplements

Spanish black radish	1 tablet three times per day
Phosphatidylcholine	1,000 mg twice per day
Lipoic acid	300 mg per day
Omega-3s	1,000 mg twice per day
Aqueous selenium	400 mcg per day
Probiotics	16 billion per day
Garlic	1 capsule per day (should contain 1 bulb per capsule)
MSM	2,000 mg per day

Nutritional Approaches

Work with a nutritionally oriented physician to get your mercury levels checked. If your levels are high, it might be necessary to undergo chelation therapy. It is helpful to monitor your levels on an annual basis. Cook with cilantro, which naturally chelates mercury. Try it as a base for pesto sauce. Eat as cleanly as possible, with plenty of protein, whole grains, and dark green leafy vegetables, which will give your body the support it needs to eliminate mercury. Incorporate wild Alaskan salmon, sardines, and halibut (from www.vitalchoice.com) into your diet as a clean source of fish.

PMS

Supplements

Milk thistle	300 mg per day
Calcium	500 mg twice per day on an empty stomach
Magnesium	400–800 mg on an empty stomach
Inositol	1 teaspoon of powder mixed into water, up to six times per day
Chaste tree	4 tablets per day (from *Vitex agnus-castus* fruit; 500 mg)
St. John's wort	1 teaspoon of liquid tincture (from *Hypericum perforatum* flowering herb 2.5 g)
Omega-3s	2,000 mg per day
Borage oil	500 mg per day

Nutritional Approaches

Each menstrual cycle, some femmes feel more fatale thanks to a unique form of physical torture: PMS. Chaste tree helps keep hormones balanced by promoting healthy progesterone levels and sustaining regular menstrual cycles. Make sure you eat enough protein and dark green leafy vegetables throughout the day, especially the week before your period. Be mindful of St. John's wort and chaste tree if you take the pill; about 1 percent of the population has a decrease in contraceptive efficacy. For bad PMS, plunk yourself down in an Epsom salts bath. Also, hustle on over to a yoga class, or pop in a yoga DVD at home. Yoga does wonders for leveling out your hormones.

POLYCYSTIC OVARIAN SYNDROME

Supplements

Chromium picolinate	500 mcg twice per day
Lipoic acid	300 mg twice per day
Omega-3s	3,000 mg per day
Evening primrose oil	1,000 mg per day
Vitamin D	2,000 IU per day

Nutritional Approaches

PCOS is linked to insulin resistance, so avoid sugar. Eat as balanced a diet as you can, and trade in sugary sodas for flavored seltzers. Try sweetening your foods with agave syrup or stevia powder, both of which are naturally low in sugar and chemical-free. Avoid high-fructose corn syrup like the plague!

QUITTING SMOKING

Supplements

Licorice root	(from *Glycyrrhiza glabra* root 2.5 g) First thing in the morning, take 1 teaspoon of liquid tincture diluted in 1 ounce of water
Tyrosine	1,000 mg per day
5-HTP	100 mg per day
Vitamin C	500 mg three times per day
B-complex vitamins	50 mg per day

Nutritional Approaches

When you initially quit smoking, you may find that you crave sugar like crazy, because your blood sugar will be all over the road map for the first few months. To help your body adjust, try adding green vegetable juices to your diet a few times per week. They will pump your insides with hundreds of vitamins and minerals and help your lungs and adrenal glands heal and recover, which will ultimately stabilize your mood and your cravings. Also try keeping a bottle of lavender essential oil handy; a few dabs on your wrist a few times a day will help promote relaxation.

STOMACH ULCERS

Supplements

L-glutamine	3,000 mg of powder diluted in water, three to six times per day
DGL	760 mg, three times per day between meals
Probiotics	8 billion, twice per day with meals
Slippery elm tea	Mix 1 teaspoon of powder to a paste with cold water. Slowly add a cupful of hot water while whisking, otherwise you will get lumps. Pour into a cup and add a little honey, if desired. The consistency will be like a thick porridge. Have 3 cups per day.

Nutritional Approaches

If you're a coffee junkie you'll need to go cold turkey until well after your stomach is healed, otherwise, you'll just be pouring more acid into your stomach, making your symptoms worse. Prepare yourself for battle by brewing pitchers of peppermint or chamomile tea. Tomatoes and citrus may be irritating to your stomach; keep a food diary and be mindful of what works for you. Make sure you eat plenty of protein to heal your stomach, as well as carbs that are easy to digest: pineapple and papayas, sweet potatoes, brown rice, slow-cooked oats, winter squash, and vegetable soups.

SUGAR CRAVINGS

Supplements

Lipoic acid	300 mg per day
Calcium	500 mg twice per day
Magnesium	400 mg twice per day
Zinc	25 mg per day
Aqueous selenium	200 mcg per day
Tyrosine	500 mg twice per day on an empty stomach; you can take up to 2,000 mg per day if needed
5-HTP	300 mg per day
L-glutamine	5,000 mg per day in powdered form, mixed into water

Nutritional Approaches

It can take your body up to seven days to eliminate sugar from your system, so try to go cold turkey. (Once you're over the hump, it does get easier, I promise!) It's very important to eat small, frequent meals throughout the day to stabilize your blood sugar. Snack on raw nuts and seeds, which are rich in trace minerals that will help curb cravings. Also, avoid diet sodas and artificial sweeteners and allow some time for your taste buds to learn a new way of living; you're better off using agave syrup or stevia powder, or even a little maple syrup or honey.

THINNING HAIR

Zinc	25 mg per day
Magnesium	400 mg per day
Hyaluronic acid	150 mg per day
N-acetyl cysteine	1,000 mg per day
Omega-3s	2,000 mg per day
Evening primrose oil	1,000 mg per day

Nutritional Approaches

Chicken stock made from bones is naturally rich in hyaluronic acid, and root vegetables like sweet potatoes are naturally rich in magnesium, so feel free to incorporate both into your diet. Your local health-food store is a valuable resource for premade organic chicken stock, and I like to cook brown rice in the stock for a yummy risotto. Medically, make sure you get your thyroid checked; an under- or overactive thyroid can be a cause for thinning hair. In addition, stress can cause hair loss, so take a minute to reflect on what's been happening in your life in the past six months or so.

THYROID (LOW)
BMR (Basal Metabolic Rate) Test

This test determines your thyroid function using your basal body temperature—your body's temperature at rest. If your thyroid is running low, your body's temperature drops below normal while you're at rest or asleep.

Perform the test by measuring your underarm temperature upon waking in the morning. For accuracy, perform the test five mornings in a row, and then calculate the average. Do not perform this test during ovulation (usually days eleven through fourteen of your monthly cycle); your body temperature may be falsely elevated during that time.

1. The night before, shake down an oral glass thermometer and set it in a safe place next to the bed.
2. Immediately upon waking, without raising your head from the pillow, place the thermometer under one armpit.
3. Leave the thermometer under your arm for 10 minutes.
4. Move as little as possible during the process and try to remain flat on your back, otherwise the thyroid gland will be activated and you'll get a false reading.
5. After 10 minutes, remove the thermometer and record the temperature.

If your temperature falls below 97.8 degrees, visit your nutritionally-oriented doctor ASAP!

URINARY TRACT INFECTIONS (UTIs)

Supplements

D-mannose

Day 1 of an active UTI: ½ level teaspoon (1 g of D-mannose) diluted in 6 ounces of water, every 2 hours, 8 A.M.–8 P.M.

Day 2: ½ level teaspoon diluted in 6 ounces of water, every 3 hours, 8 A.M.–8 P.M.

Day 3: ½ level teaspoon diluted in 6 ounces of water, every 4 hours, 8 A.M.–8 P.M.

For maintenance: ½ teaspoon daily diluted in 6 ounces of water.

To prevent "honeymoon cystitis," take 1 teaspoon of powder one hour prior to boom-boom and then again immediately afterward.

Vitamin C	1,000 mg per day. Use the ascorbic acid form of vitamin C, which can help acidify the urine and discourage bacterial growth.
Probiotics	8–16 billion per day, in either powdered or capsule form with meals

Nutritional Approaches

Cranberry products are well known for their incredible capacity to fight UTIs. In addition to acidifying the urine, cranberries contain substances that inhibit bacteria from attaching to the bladder lining and, ultimately, promote the flushing out of bacteria with the urine stream. Here's the catch: Sugar will feed the bacteria that cause UTIs, so use only lip-puckering, unsweetened cranberry juice, cranberry extract capsules, or naturally sweet blueberries, which contain similar UTI-fighting substances.

VAGINAL DRYNESS

Supplements

Wheat germ oil	Insert a capsule into the vagina at bedtime
Evening primrose oil	1 capsule twice daily
Omega-3s	2 capsules twice daily

Nutritional Approaches

Eat a healthy, whole-foods diet rich in nutrients and trace minerals, as well as essential fatty acids. Go through your cabinets and clean out the junk fats that will disrupt your body's delicate fatty acid balance: hydrogenated oils, palm oil, vegetable oil, soybean oil, margarine, and Crisco. Instead, stock your refrigerator with flaxseed oil and flaxseeds, wild Alaskan salmon, organic olive oil, coconut oil, walnut oil, and raw nuts and seeds. These will keep you moisturized and lubricated from the inside out. Don't forget to work with a nutritionally oriented physician to get your DHEA, estrogen, and progesterone levels checked, since hormonal imbalances could also be an underlying cause of vaginal dryness.

WATER RETENTION

Supplements

Vitamin B₆	50 mg twice per day
Taurine	1,000 mg twice per day
Horsetail	1 teaspoon of liquid extract (2.5 g from *Equisetum arvense* herb) diluted in water or juice

Nutritional Approaches

Drink dandelion tea throughout the day for gentle diuretic benefits. Unsweetened cranberry juice diluted in water also provides diuretic benefits, as does eating asparagus and freshly steamed or sautéed dandelion greens.

WORKOUT RECOVERY

Supplements

Calcium	500 mg before each workout and 500 mg before bedtime
Magnesium	400 mg before each workout and 400 mg before bedtime
CoQ10	100 mg before each workout
Lipoic acid	100 mg before and after each workout
L-carnitine	1,000 mg first thing in the morning and 1,000 mg after each workout; try to take all L-carnitine before 4 P.M.
Omega-3s	1,000 mg twice per day

Nutritional Approaches

Within an hour after working out, eat a meal that combines protein, carbohydrates, and fats to replace your glycogen stores and balance your blood sugar. To prevent next-day soreness, take a warm Epsom salts bath (2 cups of salts per bath) for 20 minutes.

If you're training for an endurance event, make your own healthy sports repletion drink: 8 ounces organic juice, such as apple, grape, or pomegranate, mixed with 8 ounces water and ⅛ teaspoon sea salt. Combine all the ingredients and shake well. Store for up to twenty-four hours in the refrigerator. You can also make your own power gel: take 2 tablespoons of raw, organic honey and add one of the following: 2 tablespoons raw peanut butter, 2 tablespoons apple butter, or half a banana. Combine the ingredients and run through the blender until smooth and creamy. Add 1 teaspoon lemon juice (to cut the sweetness) and blend again. Carry during your long run in a fuel-belt bottle.

YEAST AND SINUS INFECTIONS

Supplements

Probiotics	8 billion twice per day
Garlic	1 capsule twice per day (should contain 1 bulb per capsule)
Spanish black radish	1 tablet per meal
Boric acid suppositories	600 mg boric acid suppositories inserted vaginally every night before bed for three to five nights

Nutritional Approaches

Cook with fresh garlic and coconut oil, which are natural antifungals that fight yeast. Limit your intake of sugar and sweets, yeasted foods, and foods that have trace amounts of fungus or mold: pasta, bread, sweets, mushrooms, soy sauce, vinegar, wine, and peanuts. Look out for the yeastier alcoholic drinks like wine and beer; stick to hard alcohols with a splash of club soda and lime. If you are on the pill, make sure you take 50 mg of vitamin B_6 per day. Use condoms and practice good hygiene after sex.

CHAPTER 08

GORGEOUS
in green

HOME GREEN HOME

Believe it or not, the air inside your house is more toxic than the air outside your house because of the off-gassing from carpeting, sofas, particle board, fabric softeners, and cleaning products. So, it helps to know that the simple act of keeping plants throughout your home neutralizes some of these toxic gasses and makes it a cleaner place to live. Filter your tap water to remove mercury, lead, and arsenic; water carries toxins out of our bodies so ingesting it poisoned doesn't help your body. Also, keep your home fresh with circulating air. And try to purchase green products, which not only preserve the environment, they reduce the work our bodies have to do to metabolize and detoxify chemicals present in products.

A BREATH OF FRESH AIR

Keep your home fresh with well-ventilated, circulating air (think ceiling fans and cracking open the windows). Consider a HEPA filter to purify the air if you live in an urban environment or have high amounts of air pollution outside your home.

If you regularly suffer from nosebleeds brought on by dry air, invest in a humidifier. Cool-mist humidifiers don't boil water, so they are safer and more energy-efficient than warm-mist humidifiers. Also, look for brands that contain ionic silver sticks, which prevent microbial growth. Be sure to clean your humidifier with hot, soapy water at least once per week, and soak the base with white vinegar to kill any funky buildup present. For a poor-man's humidifier that is also ecofriendly, plunk down a bowl of fresh water on the radiator before bed. Heat plus moisture equals humidity. *Sayonara* sore throats, hello dewy skin!

YOU CAN LEAD A GAL TO WATER

Filter your tap water to remove mercury, lead, arsenic, and crypto-sporidium. Since water has the almighty job of carrying toxins out of our bodies, we need to do our best to make sure it is clean.

Drinking water has become a bit of a conundrum. Staying well hydrated is key to keeping Gorgeous, but all those plastic bottles we buy are petroleum-based and don't always get recycled. All of a sudden, a good habit becomes bad for the environment. And keep this in mind: The Natural Resources Defense Council conducted an in-depth assessment of tap versus bottled water and concluded that, while much tap water is risky to drink, bottled water is not necessarily any safer.

So how do we preserve both our health and the Earth's? The best way to get your internal pipes cleaned is with a home water purification system. It's the most economical, convenient, and effective way of getting high-quality, healthy water. Be sure to think about shower filters as well; we take in as much, or more, chemicals through our skin as we do orally.

THE FLUORIDE CONTROVERSY

Fluoride is a very controversial topic. There are numerous substantiated studies showing direct toxic effects (brain damage, increased risk of cancer) of fluoride on the body. Although the natural form of fluoride is part of the composition of your teeth, ingesting it orally is a problem. The good news is that you can look to your diet for naturally healthy teeth. Keeping sugar low on your dietary list and diving head-first into a whole foods diet are surefire ways to keep your teeth healthy naturally. You can also protect yourself by using fluoride-free toothpaste and talking to your dentist about using nonfluoride fillings or bonding materials. Pitcher and faucet filters won't remove fluoride effectively, but installing a reverse osmosis filter will do the trick.

At present, the American Dental Association and the National Research Council have both raised serious concerns about the safety of fluoridated water for infants and young children, as the addition of fluoride to water is dangerous for children. Exposure to 4 mg of fluoride per liter—the EPA's maximum allowable concentration—can cause severe tooth enamel fluorosis and increased risk for bone fractures with lifelong consumption.

CLEAN AND GREEN

Today's cleaning products are definitely stronger than your momma's elbow grease, but they often contain a plethora of chemicals that raise health and environmental concerns. No law requires manufacturers of cleaning products to list ingredients on their labels or to test their products for safety, so let's all hold hands, sing "Kumbaya," and make sure that our homes are not only clean but nontoxic, too! Baking soda, salt, and vinegar can clean just about anything in your home and won't make you sick, either. For safe household products, pick up Seventh Generation, Mrs. Meyer's, or Method cleaning products.

GREEN SWEEP

For you DIYers who like to take matters into your own hands, try these natural cleaners. They are cost-effective and extremely safe:

All-purpose cleaner. Mix ½ cup vinegar and ¼ cup baking soda into ½ gallon water. Use to clean countertops, shower stall panels, bathroom mirrors, windows, and chrome fixtures.

Dishwashing soap. Use liquid soap and add 2 tablespoons white vinegar to warm, soapy water for tough jobs.

Toilet bowl cleaner. Mix ¼ cup baking soda and 1 cup vinegar. Pour into toilet bowl and let it set for a few minutes. Scrub with brush and rinse.

GLASS ACT

Now I hate to be all Debbie Downer here, but in the name of food safety and hormonal balance, it's time to toss out plastic. I know, I know—it's a tough battle negotiating the delicate balance of convenience versus health benefits when it comes to plastic in our day-to-day lives.

But here's the deal with plastic: Plastic contains Bisphenol A, an estrogen agonist that activates estrogen receptors, mimicking the effects of estrogen in the body. This can lead to breast and uterine cancer in women, decreased testosterone levels in men, and it can also have very dangerous effects on babies and young children. To play it safe, keep glass water bottles on hand that you can reuse—the Voss ones are particularly sexy. Also, check out Sigg Swiss-engineered aluminum drinking bottles, which are reusable and safe. Try not to refill plastic water bottles, unless they are the thicker Nalgene bottles, which are less likely to leach plastic compounds into your water. Store leftover food in the fridge in ceramic or glass containers. Never use plastic in the microwave; heat your food in a glass container or on a plate.

BE A LOCAVORE

While most of us will never physically own our own farms, we can certainly support our dear farmers by purchasing locally grown and sustainably harvested foods. Sustainable harvesting ensures that we can use renewable resources while guaranteeing that they and their environment continue to thrive indefinitely. This ultimately improves farmers' lives by creating a transparent and sustainable food supply chain—which teaches us to honor, preserve, and cooperate with nature. Bring it on! Do your part by shopping at local farmers' markets and food co-ops. You'll also be enjoying foods that are nutrient-rich because they're fresh from farm to plate.

The other benefit to buying food locally is the amount of petrol saved in transporting the foods cross-country and into our local markets. Eating just one meal per week grown locally can literally reduce our country's oil consumption by more than one million barrels of oil every week!

GREEN BETWEEN THE SHEETS

The same rules of gorgeous, green living can also applied in the boudoir.

Before you start your night, keep some organic lube handy so you can slip-slide away without any painful repercussions. By steering clear of petroleum-based lubes you'll be liberating yourself from your dependence on fossil fuels. (Same goes for lip balms; try beeswax-based balms instead of petroleum-based balms.)

When it comes to sex toys, be mindful of plastic-based paraphernalia. Many store-bought sex toys are rich in phthalates, a chemical compound used to make products soft and flexible. Phthalates can mimic the effects of estrogen and ultimately lead to hormonal disruption, so go for glass, metal, silicone, elastomers, or hard plastic trinkets instead, which will give a whole new meaning to safe sex. And if you're using battery-operated devices, just use rechargeable batteries, you little Energizer Bunny!

Other ways you can save energy and have fun: Take a power shower for two, buy organic cotton or bamboo sheets, use energy-efficient light bulbs in the bedroom, and use all-natural organic and pure massage oils. Giving back to the Earth never felt better!

GORGEOUS
glossary

5-HTP (5-Hydroxytryptophan): 5-HTP is an amino acid that is the intermediate step between tryptophan and the important brain chemical serotonin. In this stress-filled era, the lifestyle and dietary practices of many people can cause lower levels of serotonin within the brain. As a result, many people are overweight, crave sugar and other carbohydrates, experience bouts of depression, get frequent headaches, and have vague muscle aches and pain. All of these maladies are correctable by raising brain serotonin levels; 5-HTP facilitates this process.

A-F betafood: A-F betafood is a complex of carrots, beet juice, vitamins A and B_6, and betaine. These nutrients work synergistically to aid in the transport of fats and promote healthy liver function. A-F betafood also promotes the healthy release of bile acids, facilitating the breakdown of fats in the digestive tract.

Andrographis: *Andrographis paniculata* herb is used to support healthy upper respiratory tract function. Double-blind, placebo-controlled clinical trials support the traditional use of andrographis. It is especially effective at reducing fevers and supporting lung health when used in conjunction with echinacea and holy basil.

Aqueous selenium: Selenium is an essential trace mineral that has powerful antioxidant effects in the body. Selenium is also necessary for efficient energy production in the cell's furnace, the mitochondria, and for optimal functioning of the immune system. Aqueous selenium is particularly useful in treating mercury toxicity.

Ashwagandha root: Used in Ayurvedic medicine, and sometimes called "Indian ginseng," this herb is native to India and Africa. Ashwagandha contains compounds called withanolides, which are similar to the active constituents in ginseng. Ashwagandha helps the body adapt better to environmental stresses, enhances immune function, and promotes an overall feeling of well-being.

Astaxanthin: Astaxanthin is the red algae that wild salmon eat; it is actually what gives the salmon their pink color. Taking astaxanthin in supplement form has been proven in multiple studies to prevent hyperpigmentation and residual sun spots on the surface of the skin.

Astragalus root: Astragalus is a Chinese herb used to boost the immune system and reduce the adverse effects of stress and fatigue. It helps raise the white blood cell count and fight chronic viruses but should not be used if you have an acute infection or a fever.

Betaine hydrochloride: Betaine hydrochloride is an acidic form of betaine, a vitamin-like substance found in grains and other foods. Betaine hydrochloride is recommended by some doctors as a supplemental source of hydrochloric acid for people who have a deficiency of stomach acid (hypochlorhydria). Gastric acid is produced by the parietal cells of the stomach to ward off bacterial and parasitic intestinal infections and to digest protein properly. If you are passing a lot of stinky gas, this is for you!

Borage oil or GLA (gamma linoleic acid): GLA is the active ingredient found in the oil of borage seeds. It is an essential fatty acid in the omega-6 category, but unlike the unhealthy omega-6 oils, such as vegetable oil, borage oil has tremendous health-promoting effects. It is essential for smooth, healthy skin and helps women with hormonal balance, easing conditions such as PMS and menopause. GLA has been researched for its ability to relieve PMS, reduce inflammation caused by arthritis, lower cholesterol, and help reverse diabetic neuropathy.

Boswellia: Boswellia is an herb with anti-inflammatory benefits. It helps relieve joint pain, Crohn's disease, ulcerative colitis, and asthma. Boswellia also helps detoxify the joints, which often act as reservoirs for environmental toxins and stress.

Calcium lactate: There is more calcium in the human body than all of the other minerals combined. Your body needs it every day, not just to keep your bones and teeth strong over your lifetime, but to ensure the proper functioning of your muscles and nerves. It even helps your blood to clot. Calcium lactate is a very absorbable form of calcium.

Chaste tree: Chaste tree promotes a natural, healthy balance within the female endocrine system, supports female reproductive health, and eases temporary feelings of tension associated with the menstrual cycle. Chaste tree berries normalize irregular menstrual periods and relieve PMS symptoms such as bloating, breast tenderness, and moodiness. *Gorgeous Girl beware! DO NOT take chaste tree if you are on the pill.*

Chromium picolinate: Chromium is an essential trace mineral that is vital for blood sugar regulation and energy production. It's important in processing carbohydrates and fats, and it helps cells respond properly to insulin—the hormone produced in the pancreas that makes blood sugar available to the cells as our basic fuel. It is therefore a key nutrient for people with diabetes, high triglycerides, and insulin resistance.

Collinsonia root: Collinsonia root has long been known to support the "vascular tone" of the peripheral circulatory system. Collinsonia root also helps maintain healthy function of the kidneys. It is of reputed value in treating varicose veins and hemorrhoids.

DGL: Deglycyrrhizinated licorice is a remarkable medicine for peptic ulcers. It is extremely safe and cost-effective and is free of the side effects often seen while taking ulcer medications. The tablets must be chewed and mixed with saliva for best results. Taking DGL daily can heal an ulcer in six to twelve weeks.

DIM (Diindolylmethane): DIM, a naturally occurring phytonutrient found in cruciferous vegetables, works by increasing the body's production of the beneficial forms of estrogen, while decreasing the two forms of bad estrogen that are linked to tumor growth. DIM is an excellent therapy for treating uterine fibroid tumors, fibrocystic breasts, and the symptoms of hormonal imbalance.

DMAE (Dimethylaminoethanol): A compound found in high levels in anchovies and sardines, DMAE enhances cognitive function; small amounts of it are also naturally produced in the human brain. It increases levels of the neurotransmitter acetylcholine in the brain, making it beneficial for improving short-term memory and concentration.

D-mannose: Studies suggest that D-mannose is ten times more effective than cranberries in dislodging *E. coli* bacteria from the bladder wall and, as such, can ameliorate more than 90 percent of UTIs in twenty-four to forty-eight hours.

D-mannose is a naturally occurring sugar similar in structure to, but metabolized differently from, glucose (a component of table sugar). Because the body metabolizes only small amounts of D-mannose and excretes the rest in the urine, it doesn't interfere with blood sugar regulation, even in diabetics.

The cell wall of the UTI-causing *E. coli* bacteria has tiny fingerlike projections that contain complex molecules called lectins on their surfaces. These lectins act as a cellular glue that binds the bacteria to the bladder wall so that they cannot be readily rinsed out by urination. However, because D-mannose molecules will glom on to these lectins and fill up all of the bacterial anchoring sites, the bacteria can no longer attach to the bladder wall and are, therefore, flushed away. In other words, unlike antibiotics, D-mannose does not kill any bacteria, whether they are good or bad, but simply helps displace them.

Echinacea: Echinacea is an herb that works to both prevent and treat allergies, colds, and flus; support a weakened or suppressed immune system; and help with post-viral syndromes. Contrary to popular belief, it is safe for long-term use. Gargling with liquid echinacea can resolve a sore throat or swollen glands within twenty-four hours if used at the first signs of the symptoms. It should make your tongue feel numb, which lets you know you're using a product with active ingredients. It will also make you cough and sputter as if you've taken a straight shot of whiskey!

Evening primrose oil: Evening primrose oil is derived from the seeds of the evening-primrose plant. Like borage oil, EPO contains gamma linoleic acid (GLA) and can help relieve the symptoms of PMS, diabetes, and such inflammatory conditions as ulcerative colitis, lupus, and rheumatoid arthritis.

Folic acid: Folic acid, also called folate or folacin, is a B vitamin with a solid reputation for protecting against birth defects and heart disease. Folic acid also helps combat other ailments, such as depression, Alzheimer's disease, and certain types of cancer. Many people have a folic acid deficiency because it is easily lost through cooking or the processing of food.

Folic acid is often deficient in those who are depressed, and taking a supplement may help. Studies of depressed people with low blood levels of folic acid show that taking it in supplement form can improve the effectiveness of antidepressants. Folic acid also appears to reduce the high levels of homocysteine associated with some forms of depression.

GABA (Gamma-aminobutyric acid): GABA is the most abundant neurotransmitter in the brain. It helps induce relaxation and sleep, acting as a natural tranquilizer. GABA has also shown to be helpful in controlling seizures.

Garlic: For centuries, garlic has been recognized around the world as a spice, a food, and an herbal folk remedy. Garlic helps fight heart disease, high cholesterol, and high blood pressure. It is also a natural antibiotic and combats respiratory infections.

Goji berries: Goji berries are a sweet red fruit native to Asia. They have been used as a medicinal food for thousands of years and have been studied extensively in modern times to substantiate their health benefits. Composed of more than 15 percent protein, and with 21 essential minerals and 18 amino acids, goji berries are a nutrient-dense superfood in a class all their own.

Glutathione: Glutathione is one of the most powerful antioxidants known for its ability to protect the body against the damages caused by heavy-metal toxicity and environmental toxins. It breaks down wastes, toxins, and heavy metals into less harmful compounds. It is particularly important during acute infections, toxic-metal elimination, inflammatory bowel conditions, and all other conditions involving free-radical stress.

Glycolic acid: Glycolic acid is the smallest alpha-hydroxy acid. It is derived from sugarcane and is used topically as a skin exfoliant and moisturizer.

Horsetail *(Equisetum arvense)*: The name horsetail arose because it was thought that the plant's stalk resembled a horse's tail. Today, the most notable uses for horsetail are as a mild diuretic and as an astringent for the genitourinary system, providing relief for kidney stones and bladder infections. Scientists have even identified the compounds in horsetail that promote fluid loss (equisetonin and flavone glycosides). As a rich source of silica, horsetail is also touted for its ability to strengthen nails, hair, and teeth; the body requires silica to keep these connective tissues healthy and strong. Never take horsetail to reduce the swelling associated with poor kidney or heart function; both are potentially serious conditions that require careful medical monitoring.

Hyaluronic acid: Hyaluronic acid is a component of connective tissue whose function is to cushion and lubricate. Hyaluronan occurs throughout the body in abundant amounts. Interestingly, the availability of zinc and magnesium has an impact on hyaluronic acid levels in the body, and magnesium and zinc deficiencies are known to be associated with many of the same symptoms associated with hyaluronic acid abnormalities, such as mitral valve prolapse and poor wound healing. The jury is still out on whether hyaluronic acid is linked to breast cancer, so be sure to check with your doctor first.

Inositol: Inositol is a close relative to sugar and is part of the B-complex vitamins. One of the most versatile nutrients for promoting brain wellness, a positive and relaxed outlook, and restful sleep, inositol is also one of the most crucial nutrients for promoting female hormonal health through its role in supporting optimal liver function. Inositol also helps maintain healthy serotonin metabolism, and by so doing helps treat many conditions that involve poor serotonin function. Take the powdered form for optimal dosing.

Krill oil: Krill are tiny crustaceans found in the sea. Krill oil is a unique source of phosphatidyl choline with EPA and DHA bound to it. And because the EPA and DHA are naturally packaged inside a phospholipid, krill oil is a faster and more effective delivery of omega-3s in the body—especially to the brain. Krill oil is also a rich source of astaxanthin.

L-carnitine: L-Carnitine is a nutrient that facilitates the body's ability to burn fats for energy. Optimizing carnitine levels has been found to have dramatic benefits for combating low energy, obesity, and fatigue. Controlled trials have demonstrated that carnitine increases weight loss by promoting optimal fat burning by the mitochondria. Carnitine also helps promote heart health, maintenance of healthy cholesterol levels, and sports endurance and recovery.

L-cysteine: L-cysteine is an amino acid that is a precursor to glutathione. It is therefore an essential nutrient for helping rid the body of toxic metals like mercury and lead.

L-glutamine: L-glutamine is a conditionally essential amino acid, which means that our body can produce it but under times of stress our needs increase. L-glutamine is the most widely used ulcer preventative in China and Japan. L-glutamine heals inflammation inside the intestinal wall and ultimately boosts immune function. It helps stop diarrhea in patients who suffer from Crohn's disease or colitis, as well as those fighting the side effects of chemotherapy. L-glutamine also helps to maintain muscle mass. Use the powdered form for optimal dosing.

Licorice root: Licorice *(Glycyrrhiza glabra)* is a flavorful herb that has been used in food and medicinal remedies for thousands of years. It helps the body adapt better to stress by supporting adrenal function. Licorice acts as a demulcent (a soothing, coating agent) to relieve respiratory ailments (such as allergies, bronchitis, colds, sore throats, and tuberculosis), stomach problems (including heartburn and gastritis), inflammatory disorders, skin diseases, and liver problems.

Lipoic acid: Lipoic acid is an antioxidant that has been extensively researched for its applications in diabetes, blood sugar metabolism, heavy-metal detoxification, liver health, hepatitis, and diabetic neuropathy. Lipoic acid helps the body produce energy, thus fighting the aging process. It also optimizes the function of the insulin receptors, making it an essential nutrient for diabetics.

L-lysine: L-lysine is an essential amino acid that cannot be manufactured by the human body; we can get L-lysine only through diet or supplementation. The human body benefits from L-lysine because it promotes absorption of calcium, which ultimately boosts immune function. Lysine is a wonderful natural remedy for people with cold sores, shingles, or genital herpes.

L-theanine: L-theanine, an amino acid naturally found in tea, promotes relaxation. L-theanine helps increase GABA production in the body, creating an alert yet totally relaxed state of mind without drowsiness. It is estimated that a heavy tea drinker (six to eight cups a day) will consume between 200 to 400 mg of L-theanine daily.

Magnesium: Magnesium is the fourth most abundant mineral in the body and is essential to good health. Approximately 50 percent of total body magnesium is found in bone; the other half is found predominantly inside the cells of tissues and organs. Magnesium helps maintain normal muscle and nerve function, keeps the heart rhythm steady, supports a healthy immune system, and keeps bones strong. Because of this, magnesium serves well as a muscle relaxant and aids in relieving muscular and menstrual cramps. Magnesium also helps regulate blood sugar levels, promotes normal blood pressure, and is known to be involved in energy metabolism and protein synthesis.

Maitake D: Maitake D-fraction, an extract from the maitake mushroom, is a bioactive compound composed of uniquely branched polymers that provide immune system and cell support. Several studies suggest that maitake D-fraction works by activating immune-system messenger cells such as macrophages and cytokines. Beta-glucan, a type of polysaccharide (string of sugar molecules) obtained from several types of mushrooms, is being studied as a treatment for cancer and as an immune-system stimulant.

Micellized vitamin A: Micellized vitamin A is the most easily absorbed form of vitamin A. It is extremely safe, even in high doses, because it bypasses the liver. Micellized vitamin A is extremely useful when you need to take a therapeutic dose of vitamin A to treat asthma, lung infections, acne, skin conditions, or immune disorders. The micellization process involves turning vitamin A into water-soluble micelles, which are ultimately much more easily absorbed across the gut wall.

MSM (methylsulfonylmethane): MSM is an organic sulfur-containing nutrient that occurs naturally in the environment and in the human body. Sulfur is necessary for the structure of every cell in the body. Hormones, enzymes, antibodies, and antioxidants all depend on it. And because the body utilizes and expends it on a daily basis, sulfur must be continually replenished for optimal nutrition and health.

N-acetyl cysteine (NAC): NAC is an amino acid and a precursor to glu-tathione, the body's most powerful antioxidant. Studies have shown that NAC can help protect against such respiratory ailments as bronchitis, bronchial asthma, emphysema, and chronic sinusitis and may even help defend against lung damage caused by the cancer-causing chemicals in cigarette smoke. NAC has also been used effectively in treating inner-ear infections. Bodybuilders report that it helps them recover faster from their workouts.

Olive leaf extract: Derived from the leaves of the olive tree, olive leaf extract is an antibacterial, antiviral, and antiparasitic substance that will help fight off the common cold, as well as active herpes outbreaks. People taking blood thinners or antibiotics should exercise caution, as olive leaf extract could reduce the efficacy of both medications. For best results, look for capsules that contain 500 mg standardized to 20 percent oleuropein.

Omega-3s: Omega-3s are essential fatty acids found in fish and fish oil. About 15 percent of the alpha linolenic acid in flaxseed oil will also convert to omega-3s in the body of a healthy person. According to the National Research Council, more than sixty health conditions have been shown to benefit from essential fatty acid supplementation. Omega-3s help reduce systemic and localized inflammation; they also treat dry skin, depression, PMS and menstrual cramps, high cholesterol and triglycerides, and poor circulation. Wild Alaskan salmon, sardines, and krill are all excellent sources of omega-3 supplements, as they are all naturally low in mercury.

Oxidative damage: Oxidative damage is a major factor in the decline of physiologic function that occurs during the aging process. Because mitochondria are a primary site of generation of reactive oxygen species, they have become a major focus of research in this area. Increased oxidative damage to mitochondrial proteins, lipids and DNA have been linked to premature aging, Alzheimer's disease, Parkinson's disease, and atherosclerosis.

Pancreatic enzymes: In order to assimilate vitamins and nutrients from our food and supplements, we must be able to digest them properly. Pancreatic enzymes are critical for the digestion of proteins, fats, and carbohydrates. If you feel gassy and bloated after meals, are regularly constipated, or feel full after eating only a small quantity of food, you're a good candidate for digestive enzymes. Studies show that the foods in the typical American diet are devoid of natural enzymes and do little to help us secrete our own production of enzymes. Taking digestive enzymes will help you digest and absorb nutrients from your food, which is a large component of overall health.

PCBs: Polychlorinated biphenyls (PCBs) are a group of toxic, carcinogenic organic compounds. PCBs are used in the manufacturing of plastics and have been demonstrated to cause a variety of serious health effects, such as cancer, as well as disruptive effects on the immune, reproductive, nervous, and endocrine systems.

Phosphatidylcholine: Phosphatidylcholine is the active ingredient in lecithin. Lecithin is a fatty substance needed for a wide variety of crucial bodily functions, such as building cell membranes and helping nutrients move in and out of cells. Phosphatidylcholine breaks down fat deposits in the body, making it valuable in the prevention of atherosclerosis and heart disease. It is also essential to the liver and helps the liver remove toxins from the body.

Phosphatidylserine: Phosphatidylserine is vital to brain cell structure and function. It plays an important role in our neurotransmitter systems and in maintaining nerve connections in the brain. Phosphatidylserine not only helps boost cognitive performance and learning ability but also helps lower cortisol levels in the body brought on by stress or over-exercising.

Physio ball: The physio ball (also called a Swiss ball) is used to help strengthen and develop the core body muscles that help to stabilize the spine. The instability of the exercise ball helps develop and train the body's natural awareness, ultimately increasing balance and stability.

Prebiotics: Prebiotics stimulate the growth of healthy microflora that populate your large intestine. When these beneficial bacteria are allowed to flourish, they help keep you healthy and strong. You need to consume plenty of prebiotics to ensure you have enough probiotics populating your gut. Apples, bananas, raw apple cider vinegar, onions, garlic, asparagus, leeks, and flaxseeds are all good sources of prebiotics.

Probiotics: Natural, "good" bacteria that live in our intestines, helping the digestive tract and immune system stay healthy, probiotics are found in most yogurts and are available in powdered or capsule form. Probiotics are most commonly sold under the names "acidophilus," "bifidus," or "lactobacillus." It is imperative to take them during and after a course of antibiotics so that you can replace what's been lost.

Prostaglandins: Prostaglandins are hormone-like substances that participate in the contraction and relaxation of smooth muscle, the dilation and constriction of blood vessels, the regulation of blood pressure, and the inflammatory processes. Prostaglandins are derived from the pro-inflammatory arachidonic acid.

Quercetin: Quercetin is a bioflavanoid, one of a group of potent nutrients that are found in plants, fruits, vegetables, teas, apples, onions, and beans. Quercetin acts to inhibit the release of histamines during allergic reactions like eczema, asthma, and hay fever.

Red yeast rice: Red yeast rice is a supplement that works like the statin drugs. It has been fermented by red yeast. When taken orally, red yeast rice lowers cholesterol and triglycerides in conjunction with a healthy diet.

Resveratrol: Resveratrol is a compound found in the skins of grapes. Often promoted as "the French paradox in a bottle," resveratrol is touted as an antioxidant, an anti-cancer agent, and a phytoestrogen. It is useful in treating diseases of the blood vessels, heart, and liver.

Spanish black radish: An herb that belongs to the phytonutrient-rich cruciferous family of vegetables, Spanish black radish has a natural anti-biotic action and promotes systemic cleansing by activating the liver's primary detoxification mechanism.

St. John's wort: The herb St. John's wort is beneficial in treating mild to moderate depression, seasonal affective disorder, mild anxiety, insomnia, stress, and viral infections such as herpes, chicken pox, and shingles. Check with your doctor before taking St. John's wort if you are on any type of prescription medication, and avoid excessive sunlight. Liquid tinctures of St. John's wort will be absorbed most effectively.

Taurine: Taurine is a conditionally essential amino acid, which means the body can make it but will require more under times of stress. Vegetarians who do not eat meat will need to supplement with taurine. It serves to protect the heart and lower blood pressure, and it also helps bile acids in the gallbladder clear cholesterol from the body. Taurine works in conjunction with vitamin B_6 as a safe diuretic that will not cause any loss or imbalance of minerals in the body.

Tea tree oil: Derived from the Australian tea tree, tea tree oil is a natural antiseptic, germicide, antibacterial, and fungicide. Many people use tea tree oil for acne, athlete's foot, cold sores, gum problems, and mosquito bites. The oils from the tea tree blend well with the skin's natural oils, so it is gentle yet effective.

Trace minerals: Trace minerals—calcium, magnesium, zinc, iron, copper, manganese, and iodine—are all required for healthy thyroid, spleen, and red blood cell functions. Trace minerals act as catalysts and cofactors in countless enzymatic processes throughout the body.

Tyrosine: Tyrosine is a nonessential amino acid synthesized in the body from phenylalanine. It helps the body produce the brain neurotransmitters epinephrine, norepinephrine, and dopamine. Tyrosine is also used to produce one of the major hormones, thyroxine, which plays an important role in controlling the metabolic rate, skin health, mental health, and growth. Tyrosine is specifically used to treat depression because it is a precursor for those neurotransmitters that are responsible for transmitting nerve impulses and are essential for preventing depression. Tyrosine may also be used as a mild appetite suppressant. Be sure to notify your doctor if you are taking tyrosine while on antidepressants, because tyrosine naturally raises dopamine levels in the brain and may decrease your need for medication.

Vitamin B_6: A water-soluble vitamin that is essential for good health, vitamin B_6 is needed for protein metabolism and red blood cell metabolism. The nervous and immune systems need vitamin B_6 to function efficiently. Vitamin B_6 is known to help naturally regulate water balance in the cells. It works in conjunction with taurine as a safe diuretic that does not cause any loss or imbalance of minerals in the body.

Vitamin D: Vitamin D is a fat-soluble steroid hormone that has long been known for its important role in regulating body levels of calcium and phosphorus and in the mineralization of bone. Vitamin D is even more important than calcium in building bone density, because it controls intestinal absorption of calcium. In addition to taking vitamin D orally, it is helpful to get fifteen minutes of sunshine three times per week to help your body make adequate amounts of vitamin D.

Wheat germ oil: Wheat germ oil is a rich source of vitamin E that is derived from the wheat berry. Vitamin E is a potent antioxidant that can help us make our sex hormones. It can be taken orally or inserted into the vagina at bedtime to relieve dryness.

Zinc: Zinc is an essential mineral that is found in almost every cell. It stimulates the activity of approximately one hundred enzymes, which are substances that promote biochemical reactions in your body. Zinc supports a healthy immune system, is essential for wound healing, helps maintain your sense of taste and smell, and is needed for DNA synthesis. Zinc is also a precursor for estrogen, progesterone, and testosterone.

index

Acknowledgments

To my A-Team of Goddesses: Celeste Fine, Jodi Warshaw, and Kate Prouty—I am blessed and lucky to work with all of you! Heartfelt thanks. Andrea Burnett, you are a PR rock star—I heart you, again and again. Yvonne Wallgren—thank you for your skintastic recipes. Jennifer Vallely, for your endlessly naughty suggestions. The Deva darlings, Sheri and Lorraine, for your t*hair*apy. And to Jeremy, for your unwavering support and for taking care of Ben so I could get this all done! My heart and soul belong to you.